IMAGES
of America

GROTON-MYSTIC EMERGENCY SERVICES

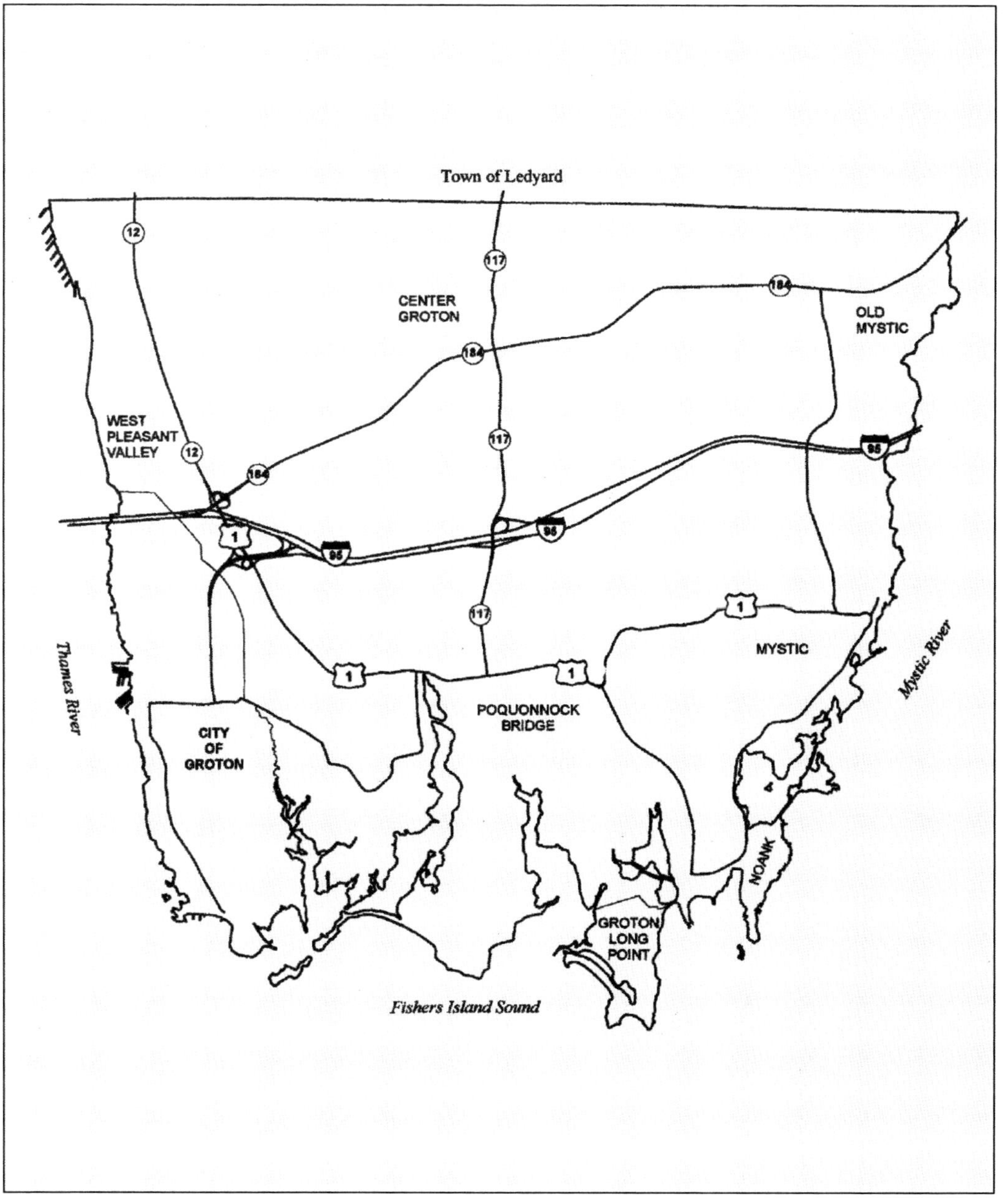

This map depicts the separate fire districts of Groton, Connecticut. (Town of Groton.)

On the Cover: On April 29, 1963, a fire, which reportedly started as a result of a faulty heating burner, destroyed the First National Food Store located on the south end of a 22-store shopping center on Long Hill Road in Groton. All area fire departments were dispatched to fight the fire, which was brought under control in about an hour. Firefighters were able to save all the remaining stores. This photograph shows three firefighters from the City of Groton Fire Department directing water into the burning building. (Jim Streeter.)

IMAGES
of America

GROTON-MYSTIC EMERGENCY SERVICES

James L. Streeter and William J. Tischer

ARCADIA
PUBLISHING

ISBN 978-1-4671-2394-5

Published by Arcadia Publishing
Charleston, South Carolina

Printed in the United States of America

Library of Congress Control Number: 2016935384

For all general information, please contact Arcadia Publishing:
Telephone 843-853-2070
Fax 843-853-0044
E-mail sales@arcadiapublishing.com
For customer service and orders:
Toll-Free 1-888-313-2665

Visit us on the Internet at www.arcadiapublishing.com

This book is dedicated to the men and women—past, present, and future—who provide the varied emergency services to our community. Whether they are paid or volunteer, these individuals have taken responsibility for the enormous task of saving and protecting the lives and property of those in our community. These individuals put their lives on the line, and their efforts often go unnoticed or are taken for granted.

The authors wish to thank each and every one of them for their efforts.

Contents

Foreword

As we take inspiration from the past we shall be vigilant in our dedication to meet the needs of our community in the future.
—Jack Welch

The emergency services that local communities have come to depend on have experienced drastic changes over the years. The days when all-volunteer departments relied on ham and bean dinners to meet their budgetary needs are long gone. Local business owners shutting their doors when the siren, horn, or phone rang and jumping into a fire truck, police car, or ambulance to respond to an emergency call is a thing of the past.

In today's world, most emergency services departments are funded 100 percent by taxes. Various social and economic factors have made it extremely difficult to recruit and retain volunteer firefighters, supernumerary police officers, and medical responders. The volume of calls handled by emergency services has skyrocketed. Mandated training requirements and standards for emergency responders have also contributed to the hiring of full-time paid employees to respond to emergency calls. We have truly evolved into a class of highly trained and educated first responders serving a much larger population with many more challenges.

If we want to continue to provide community-based emergency services, we must never forget our past and always educate the young on the rich history of the emergency services that have been provided over the years. We should try to encourage others to find the time to give back to our community, honor the men and women who came before us, and build the organizations we see in this book.

There is nothing more painful than witnessing a tragedy with loss of life or one in which someone's life has been impacted by a fire, crime, or medical emergency. On the other hand, there is no better feeling than saving a life or seeing the face of someone who has been helped by the many individuals, both paid and volunteer, who respond or who work behind the scenes for our emergency services departments. Without regret, I have dedicated the past 39 years of my life, both as a volunteer and a paid firefighter, to help my community.

This book will help keep alive the history and dedication of many people who have served—and continue to serve—in the various emergency services departments in Groton.

—Kenneth W. Richards Jr.
Fire Chief/Fire Marshal
Old Mystic Fire Department

Acknowledgments

We would like to thank the following people and organizations: Frank Bailey, Nick Brown, Everest Brustolon, Jeff Chandler, Steven Christina, Brian Connoly, Robin d'Albenes, Pat Davis, Geneva deLabry, Richard Foreman, Pat Furnbaugh, Brian Giesing, Michael Gilman, Dinah Girardi, Jay Graves, Beverly Gray, Richard Green, Dale Grenstiner, Donald Hall, Bill Hart, Glen Hathaway, Gregory T. Hudgens, Edward Johnson, John Keating, Lauren Kellogg, Ronald Kersey, Leonard Kimes, Eric Knobloch, Dick Latham, Frank Lewis, Mike Malley, Shawn McComiskey, Thomas Migliaccio Jr., James Monroe, Russell Musante Jr., Rob Palmer, Juliette Parker, William Peck, Jason Pollard, Kevin Price, Gary Rassmusen, Maurice Remillard, Joe Renda, John Santacroce, Joe Sastre, Bill Scarano, Dan Scroggins, Warren Seabury, Frank Socha, Irma Streeter, Cynthia Tischer, James Turner, Phillip Tuthill, John Varone, Catherine Young, Ed Quinlan (Center Groton), Kirsten Cohoon (Old Mystic), Chief Thomas Clapsadle, Chief Thomas Davoren, Chief Nicholas Delia, Chief Derek Fauntleroy, Chief Jeffrey Firman, Chief Louis Fusaro Jr., Chief Fritz Hilbert, Chief Tim Main, Chief Jeffrey Nixon, Chief Ken Richards, Chief David Steel, Deputy Chief Robert Tompkins, Chief Joseph Winski, Center Groton Fire Department, City of Groton Fire Department, City of Groton Police Department, Groton Ambulance Association, Groton Long Point Police Department, Groton Long Point Fire Department, Mystic Fire Department, Old Mystic Fire Department, Mystic River Ambulance Association, Noank Fire Department, Poquonnock Bridge Fire Department, Town of Groton Emergency Dispatch, Town of Groton Police Department, Groton–New London Airport, Groton Public Library, Lawrence and Memorial Hospital Paramedics, the Naval Submarine Base New London public relations office, and *The Day* newspaper.

Introduction

When it comes to providing emergency services, Groton, Connecticut, is probably one of the most unique and convoluted communities in the state of Connecticut, if not the country.

The Town of Groton, which encompasses a large portion of Mystic, Connecticut, consists of nine separate subdivisions also known as fire districts. These are the Mystic Fire District, the City of Groton, the Groton Long Point Fire District, the Poquonnock Bridge Fire District, the Old Mystic Fire District, the Noank Fire District, the West Pleasant Valley Fire District, and the Mumford Cove Association. All the districts were established through special acts approved by the Connecticut Legislature for specific purposes, such as fire protection, and all property owners in each district pay property taxes to the Town of Groton along with a special tax to their district for fire protection. Two of the districts—the City of Groton and Groton Long Point—also provide other services paid for with the taxes they levy.

With the exception of the Mumford Cove Association and the West Pleasant Valley Fire District, each district maintains their own fire department with appropriate facilities and firefighting equipment. The Noank Fire Department provides protection for the Mumford Cove Association, and the City of Groton Fire Department responds to West Pleasant Valley. The Mystic Fire District has two separate firefighting companies: the B.F. Hoxie Engine Company No. 1, Inc., and the Mystic Hook and Ladder Company. The City of Groton also has two companies: the Pioneer Hose Company No. 1 and the Eastern Point Volunteer Company No. 2.

Over the years, staffing at some of the districts' fire departments has changed from mostly volunteers to full-time paid firefighting personnel. One of the major contributing factors that accounts for the diminishing number of volunteers involves family economics wherein both parents find it necessary to work or, in some cases, one parent may work two jobs. This situation often requires one of the parents to be at home to care for the children, thus limiting time available for volunteering. Another factor affecting volunteering is the requirement of training, which must be established and maintained to be a volunteer member of a fire department. In the past, being a volunteer for a fire department was part and parcel of being a member of a special social network wherein various programs were organized by volunteers to financially assist their fire department and the community. Today, with vast and varied social organizations, the role of volunteer fire departments has immeasurably diminished.

Also located within the town of Groton are the Naval Submarine Base New London, the Groton–New London Airport, Pfizer (a large pharmaceutical facility), and the Electric Boat unit of General Dynamics (which builds nuclear submarines). All three of these entities established and maintain their own dedicated fire departments. The Submarine Base Fire Department has two separate fire stations: the Headquarters station is located on the submarine base proper, and the Vescovi Fire Station is located off base near the off-base Navy housing complex.

Groton has also been the home of four separate police departments: Town of Groton, City of Groton, Groton Long Point, and Troop E of the Connecticut State Police Department. The Avery Point Campus of the University of Connecticut, the Groton–New London Airport, Electric Boat, and the Naval Submarine Base also maintain their own police/security departments.

Since the early 1940s, there have been two separate ambulance services within Groton: the Groton Ambulance Service and the Mystic River Ambulance Association. These associations are staffed with both full-time employees and volunteers.

All of the fire, police, and ambulance departments are responsible for providing emergency services not only within their own specific districts or jurisdictions but also throughout Groton and, at times, to other locations in New London County through a mutual aid agreement or when requested.

The residential population of Groton and Mystic totals approximately 50,000; however, the influx of workers at Electric Boat, Pfizer, and the Naval Submarine Base—as well as tourists and visitors to the various attractions in both Mystic and Groton—increases the daytime population to in excess of 70,000 to 75,000 people. The variety of residential, industrial, business, and tourism demographics contributes to the complex system of providing emergency services to the region. Although the basic emergency service system in Groton seems to be very complex and convoluted at first glance, the overall operations work very well together in providing excellent emergency services to the community.

The royalties from this book will be donated to the Salvation Army, earmarked for their Mobile Canteen, which provides refreshments to emergency responders at the scene of major incidents.

One

The Fire Districts

Going back to the late 1800s and continuing until the early 1930s, eight separate and independent fire districts have been established within the Town of Groton. Seven of the districts have their own dedicated fire departments, which are equipped with appropriate firefighting equipment. These departments are operated by either full-time or volunteer personnel or a combination of both.

The seven districts that maintain their own fire departments include Center Groton, City of Groton, Groton Long Point, Mystic, Noank, Old Mystic, and Poquonnock Bridge. The West Pleasant Valley Fire District pays for and receives fire protection from the City of Groton Fire District.

The City of Groton Fire District is comprised of two fire companies: the Pioneer Hose Company No. 1 and the Eastern Point Volunteer Company No. 2. The Mystic Fire District is also comprised of two fire companies: the B.F. Hoxie Engine Company and the Mystic Hook and Ladder Company.

All the fire departments within Groton also respond to fires and other emergencies outside of their district's jurisdictional boundaries through protocols outlined in a formal mutual aid agreement.

All of Groton's district fire department personnel, both paid and volunteer, are highly trained in firefighting, rescue, and medical emergency response and perform their duties in an extremely efficient and professional manner.

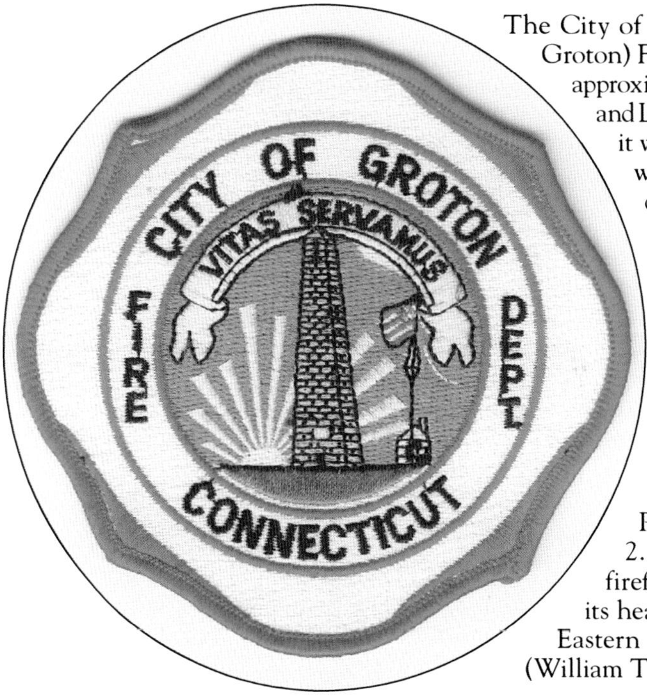

The City of Groton (formerly the Borough of Groton) Fire Department can trace it roots to approximately 1900, when the Pioneer Hook and Ladder Company was organized. When it was first established, the department was an all-volunteer organization. The department's career fire service began with the hiring of Herbert White as chief in 1920. Chief White served in that capacity for 36 years. Since then, the department has slowly and steadily grown to the current force of 17 full-time firefighting personnel. The department encompasses two volunteer companies: the Pioneer Hose Company No. 1 and the Eastern Point Volunteer Fire Company No. 2. The department also maintains firefighting equipment at two stations: its headquarters on Broad Street and the Eastern Point firehouse on Benham Road. (William Tischer.)

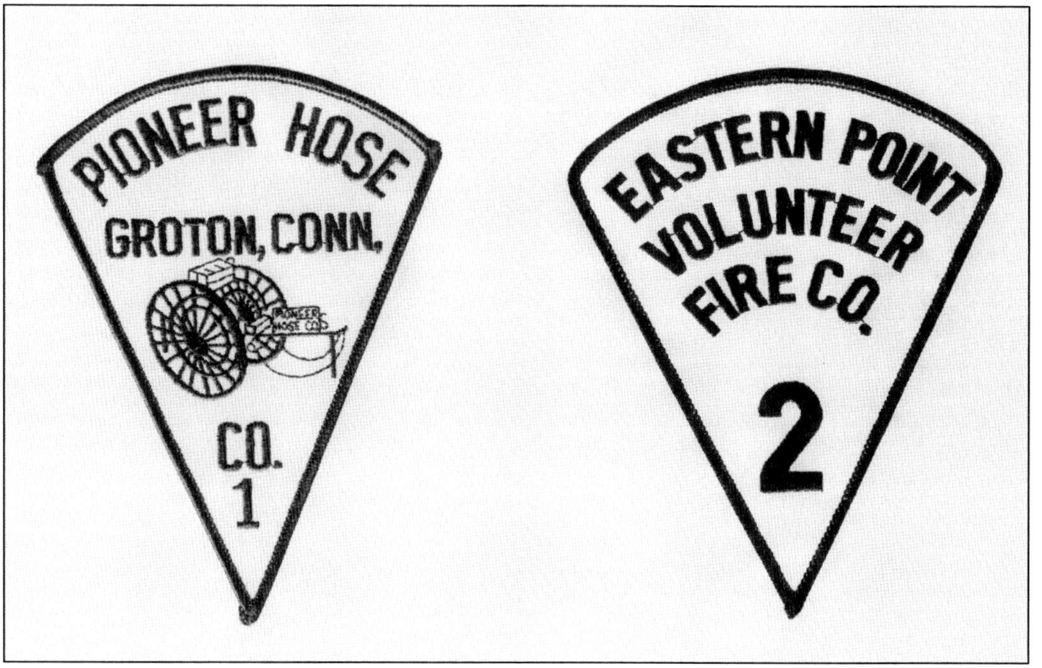

The city's volunteer companies started with the Pioneer Hook and Ladder Company in 1900. It reorganized as the Pioneer Hose Company in 1916 and moved into a station on Pleasant Street in 1917. In 1965, they relocated to the current station on Broad Street. In 1941, residents formed the Eastern Point Volunteer Fire Company in a donated house on Bill Avenue. They built a station on Benham Road in 1944 and replaced that building with the current facility in 2002. (William Tischer.)

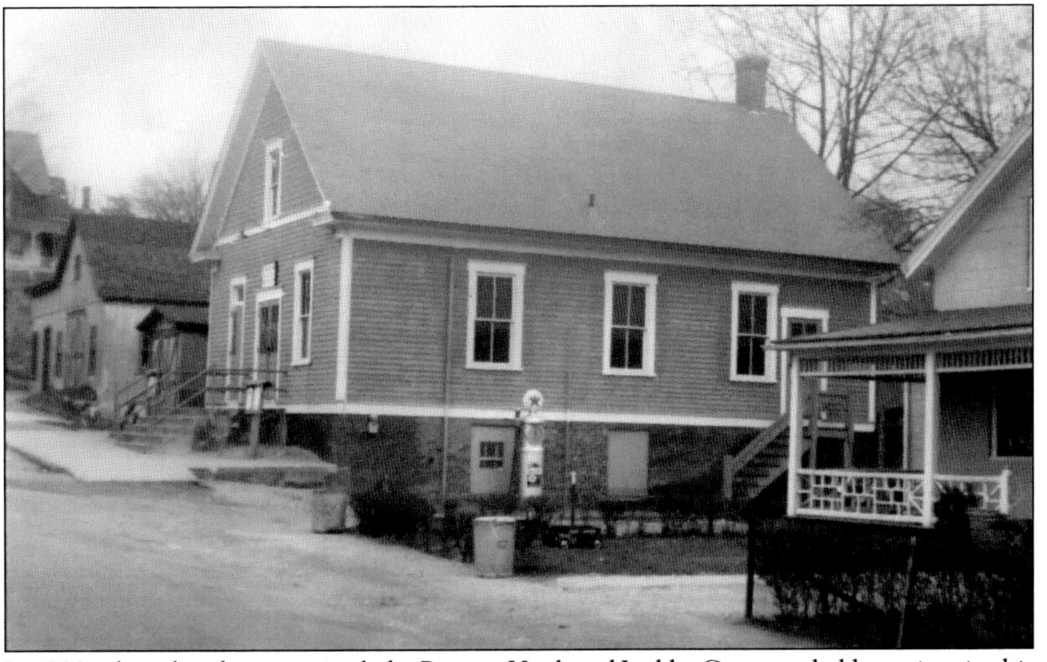

In 1900, when they first organized, the Pioneer Hook and Ladder Company held meetings in this building—the Town of Groton District 2 meetinghouse. The company's hand-drawn apparatus was stored in the basement. The building, pictured here around 1965, has been refurbished into apartments and is still in use today. (Jim Streeter.)

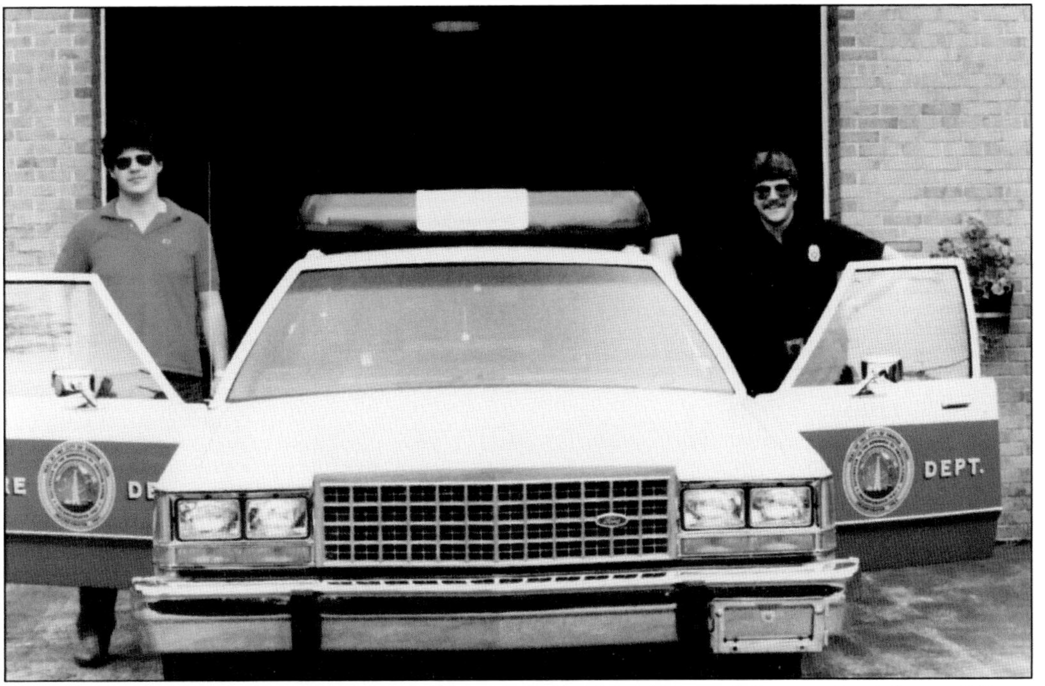

Pioneer Hose Company member Scott Blackburn (left) and City of Groton firefighter William Tischer are shown inspecting the department's new 1985 fire chief's car before it was put into service. (William Tischer.)

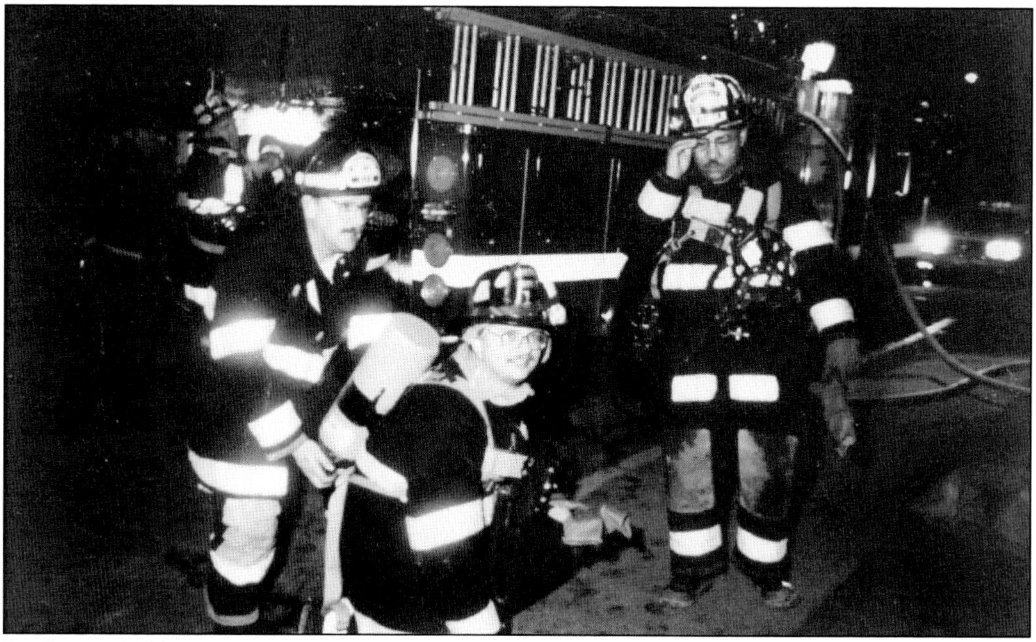

In this c. 1993 image, Pioneer Hose Company chaplain Arthur Greenleaf (left) changes an air bottle for firefighter Richard Foreman as Lt. Jonathan Gomez approaches. (City of Groton Fire Department.)

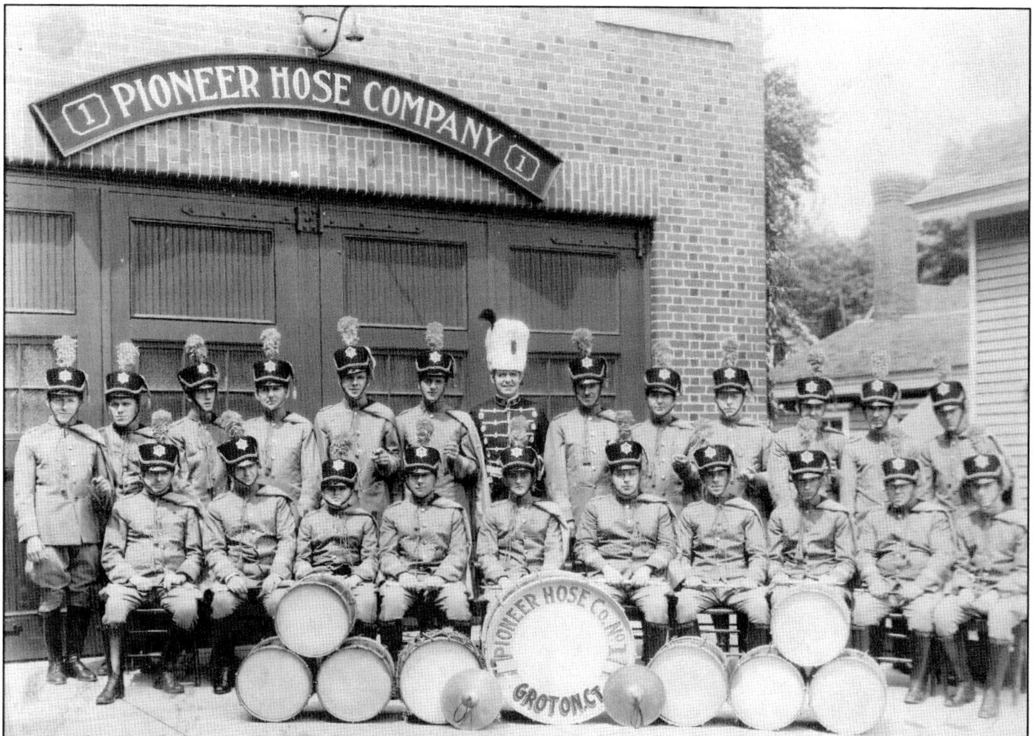

The Pioneer Hose Company Fife and Drum Band sat for this portrait during the late 1930s. In its day, the band was well known and highly regarded. (Pioneer Hose Company.)

On December 11, 1974, City of Groton deputy chief William Harmacey was leading firefighting operations on the roof of Mystic's Ancient Mariner Restaurant when he was stricken with a heart attack. Harmacey was rushed to the hospital, where he died. Deputy Chief Harmacey was 51 years old and a 20-year veteran of the department. (City of Groton Fire Department.)

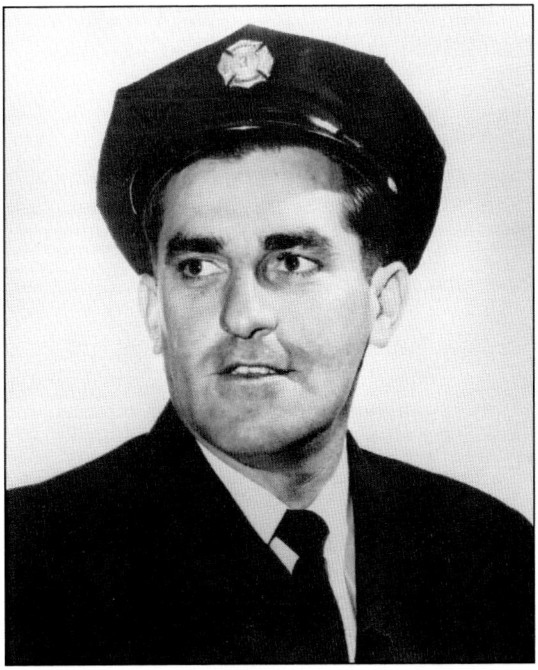

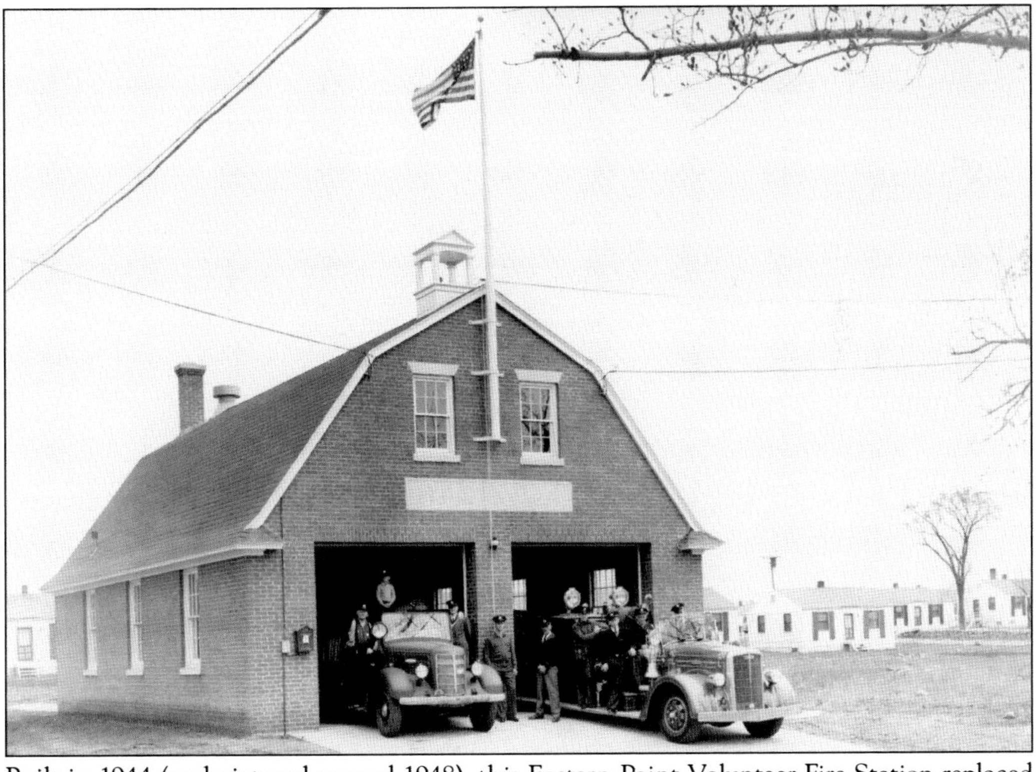

Built in 1944 (and pictured around 1948), this Eastern Point Volunteer Fire Station replaced the Bill Avenue house in which the department had been operating since 1941. The size of the building was reduced from what had been planned due to World War II restrictions. (City of Groton Fire Department.)

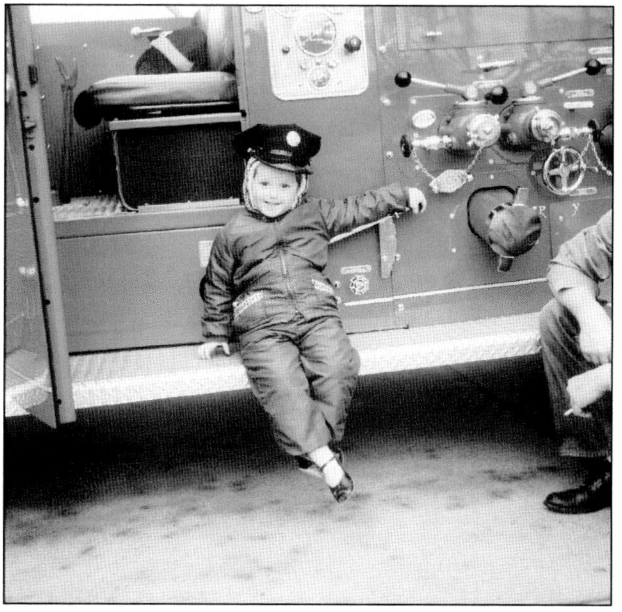

In this c. 1960 photograph, Joanne Sandora, daughter of former city police chief Joseph Sandora and niece to firefighter George Miner, hangs out with the guys. (William Scarano.)

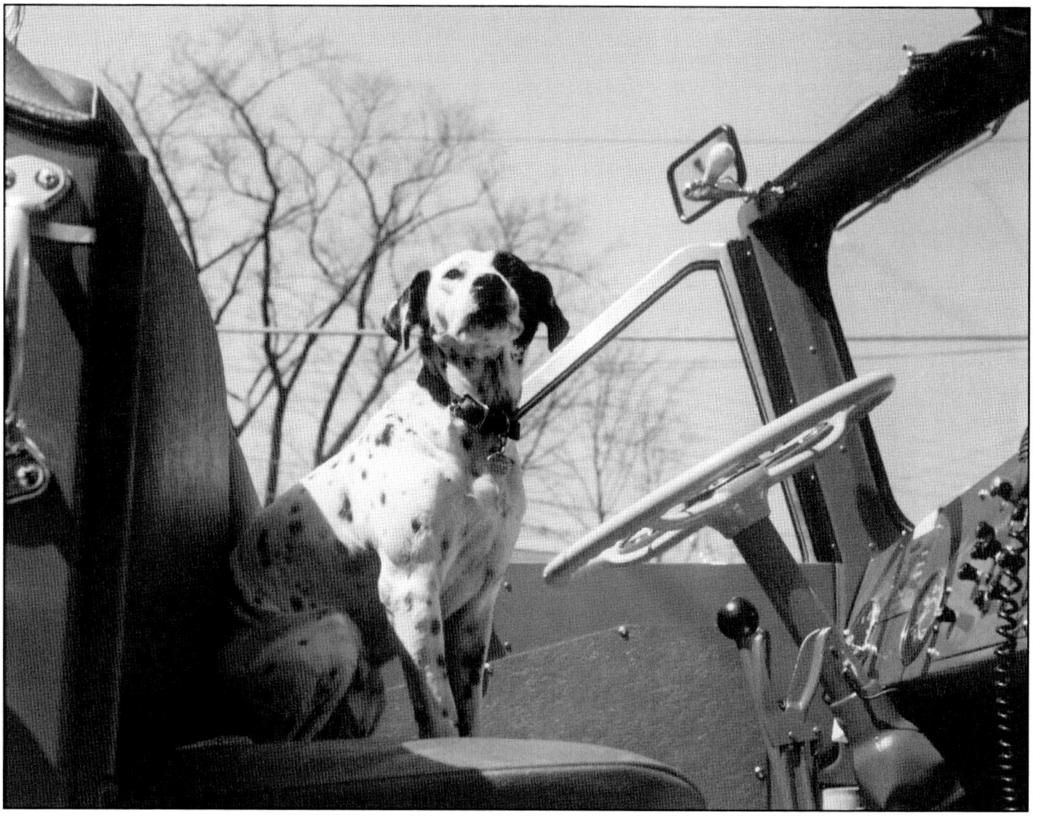

Dalmatians were part of the fire service since the horse-drawn years because of their calming effect on the horses. In this c. 1960 image, firefighter William Harmacey's dog, Spots, sits in a parked city fire truck. Apparently, Spots was afraid of running engines and often chewed on fire hoses. (William Scarano.)

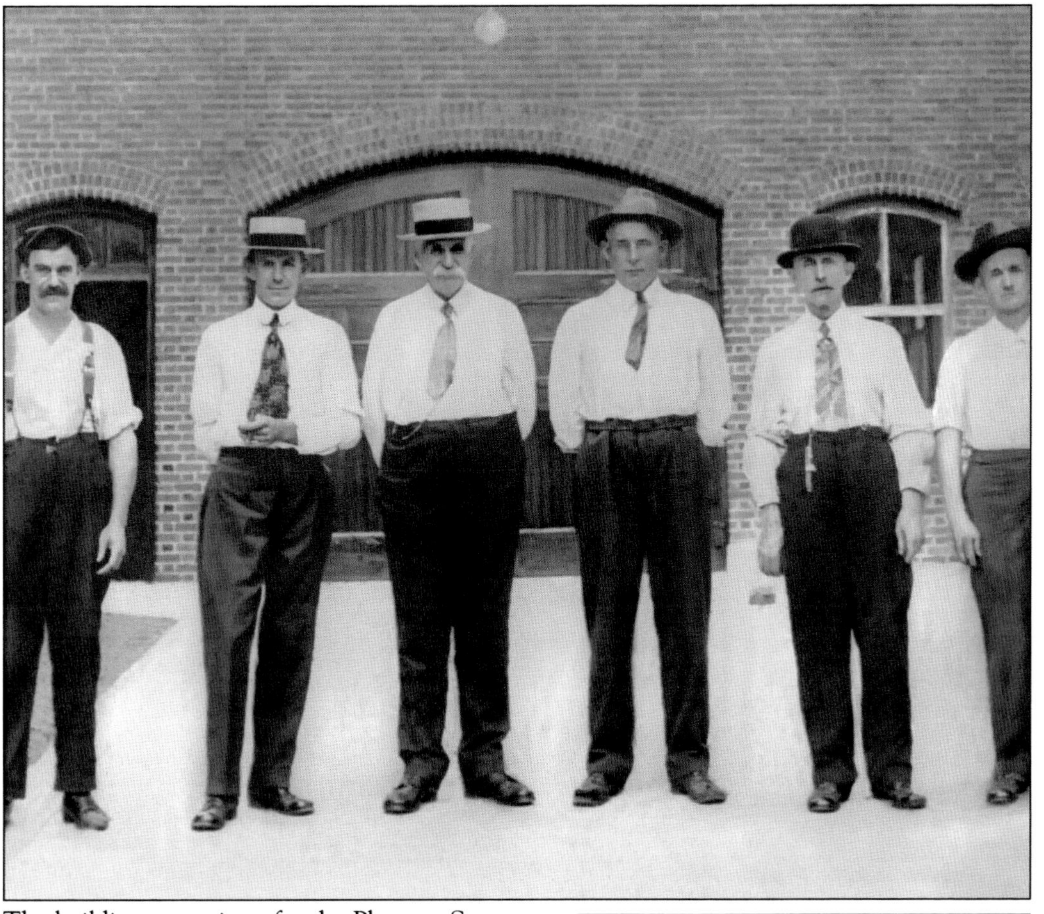

The building committee for the Pleasant Street Pioneer Hose Company fire station stands in front of the original facade in this c. 1917 picture. From left to right are William Harris, Youngs Morgan, Tyler Lamphere, William Coffin, George Hempstead, and Birt O'Fowler. (James Streeter.)

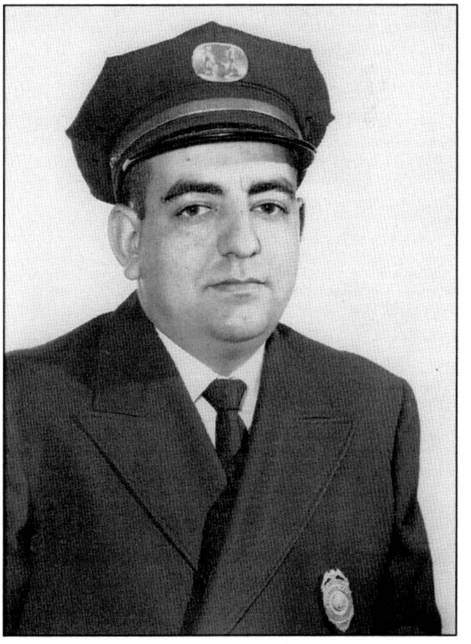

On June 25, 2000, Eastern Point Volunteer Fire Company captain Whitney C. Teehan suffered a heart attack while returning from a fire call. Teehan was rushed to the hospital, where he died. Captain Teehan was 66 years old and a 48-year veteran of the department. (Eastern Point Volunteer Fire Company.)

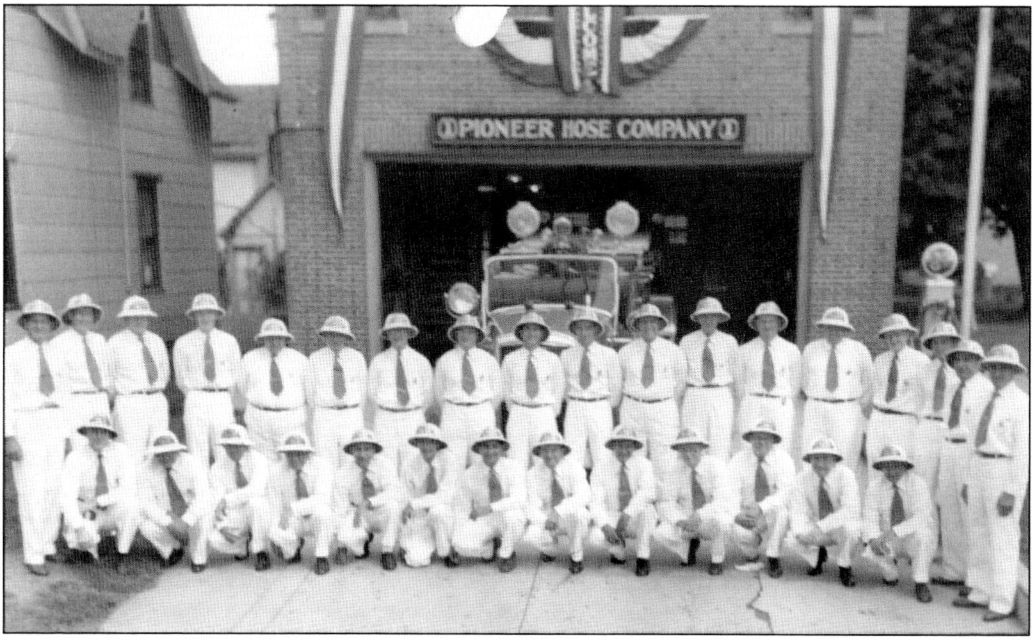

Members of the Pioneer Hose Company are pictured in the 1940s wearing white parade uniforms and pith helmets at their station. Pioneer Hose Company left the Pleasant Street station in 1965, and this building is now owned by the Merrit Graham Lodge 1871, International Association of Machinists. (Pioneer Hose Company.)

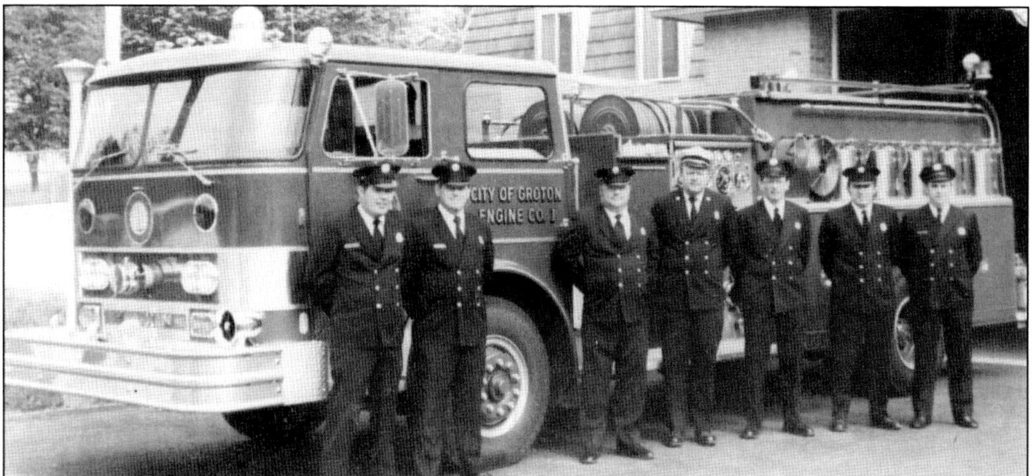

Posing with their 1973 Hahn fire engine are, from left to right, city firefighters Phillip Fogg, Leonard Kimes, Alan MacGeachie, Lt. Alan Hauser, Ellis Hartman, Donald Rollins, and John "Jack" McGrath. (Leonard Kimes Sr.)

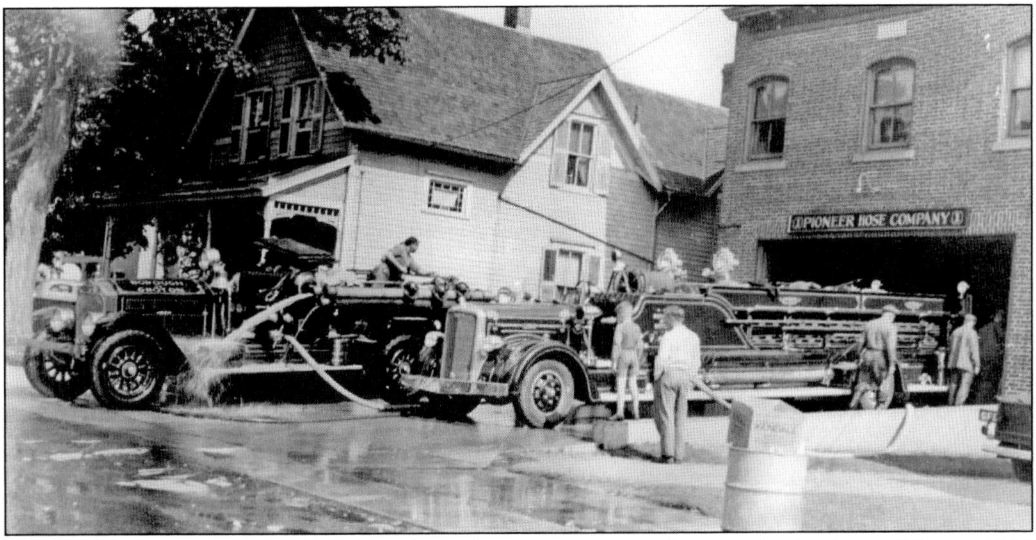

Keeping the fire apparatus clean has always been a necessary chore at the firehouse. This c. 1940 image shows Pioneer Hose Company members washing the 1927 American LaFrance engine (on the left) and the 1938 Ward LaFrance city service–type ladder truck (on the right). (Jim Streeter.)

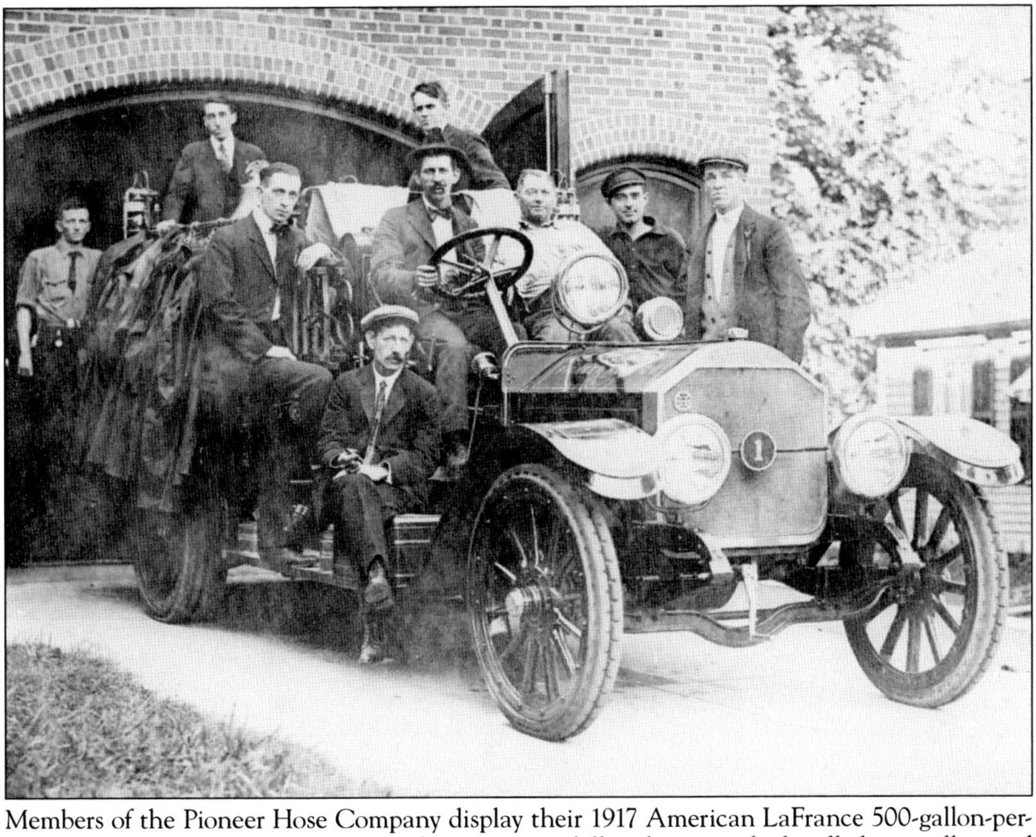

Members of the Pioneer Hose Company display their 1917 American LaFrance 500-gallon-per-minute engine in this c. 1918 picture. The "No. 1" medallion between the headlights is still owned by the company. (Pioneer Hose Company.)

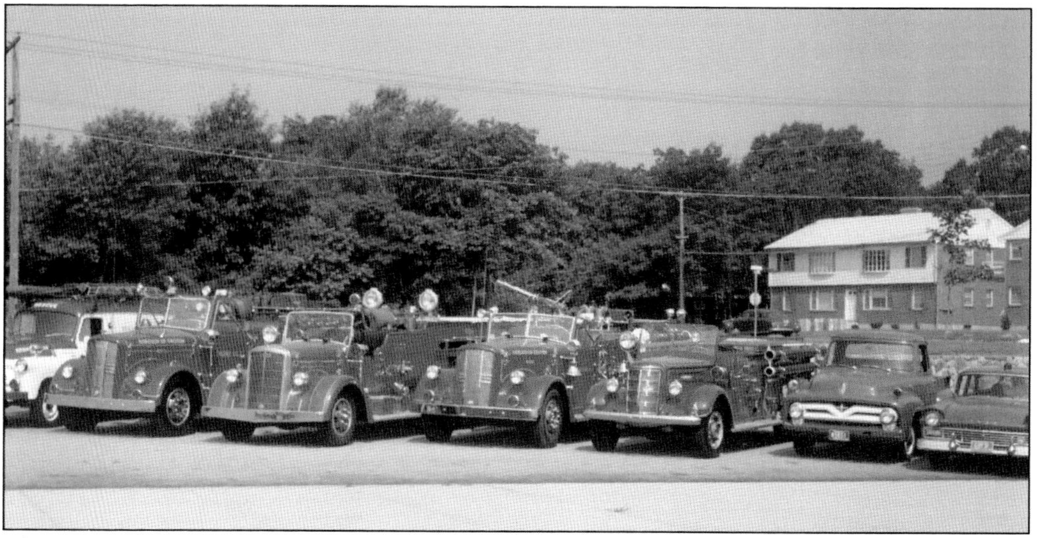

The city's firefighting fleet is shown lined up in front of West Side School on July 11, 1960. The vehicle on the far left was acquired through civil defense in 1959 and had a distinctive blue-and-white color scheme. (City of Groton Fire Department.)

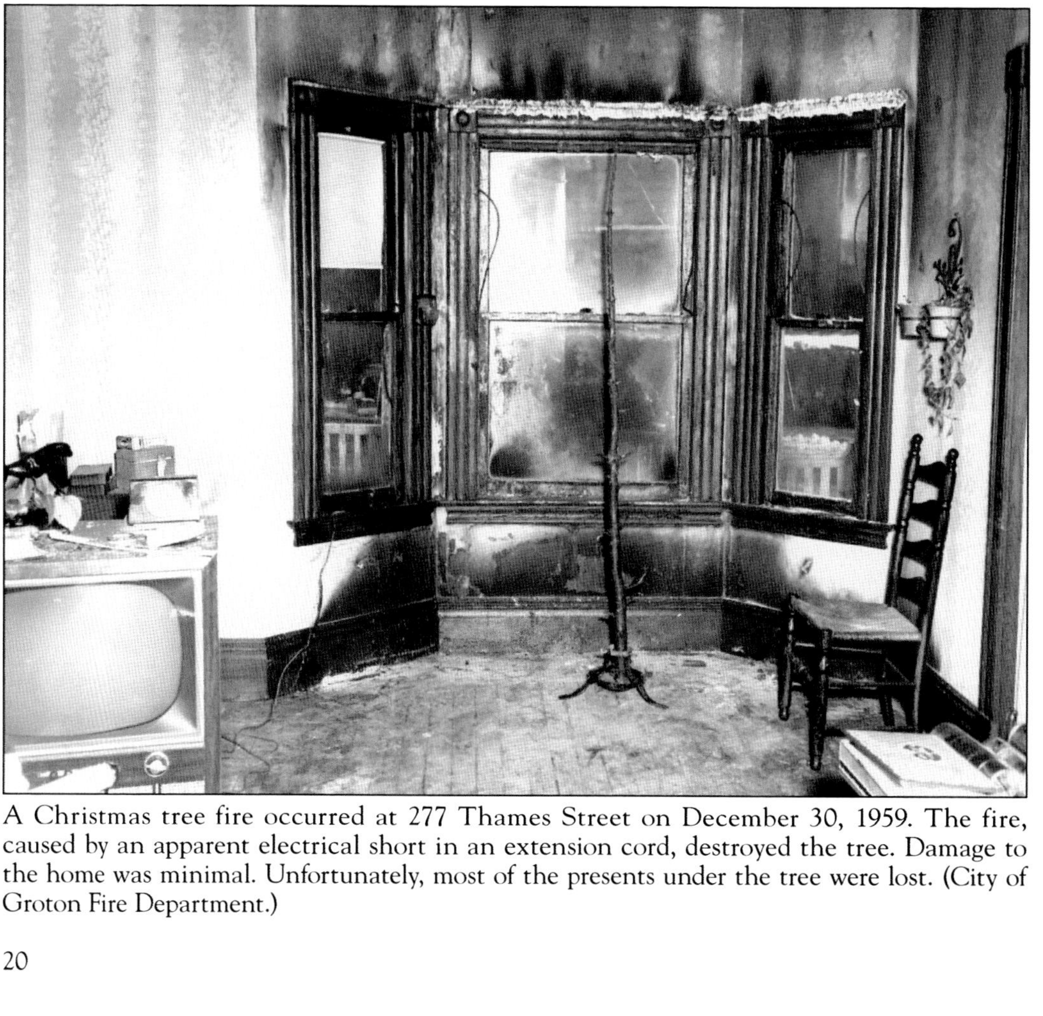

A Christmas tree fire occurred at 277 Thames Street on December 30, 1959. The fire, caused by an apparent electrical short in an extension cord, destroyed the tree. Damage to the home was minimal. Unfortunately, most of the presents under the tree were lost. (City of Groton Fire Department.)

City of Groton firefighters pose with city fire apparatus around 1960. From left to right are George Miner, Alan Hauser, William Harmacey, Erwin Newbury, Chief Raymond Fogg, William Scarano, Donald Fogg, and Wilford Landry. (William Scarano.)

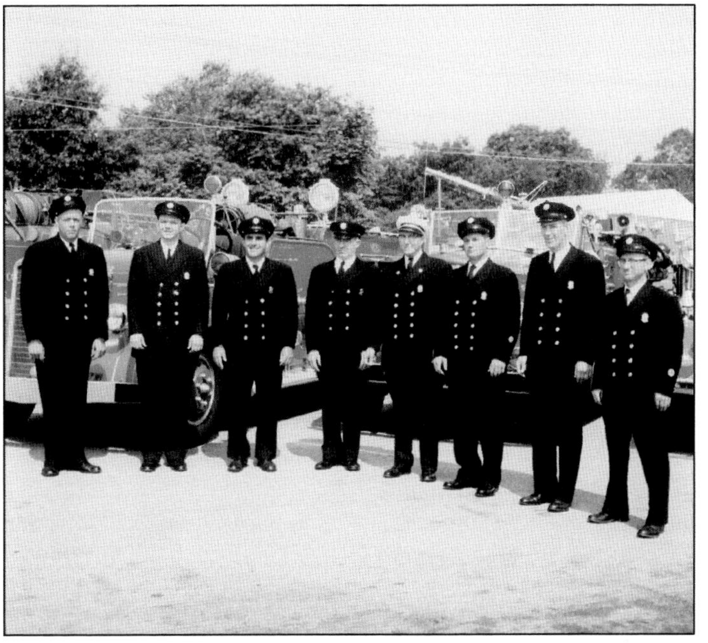

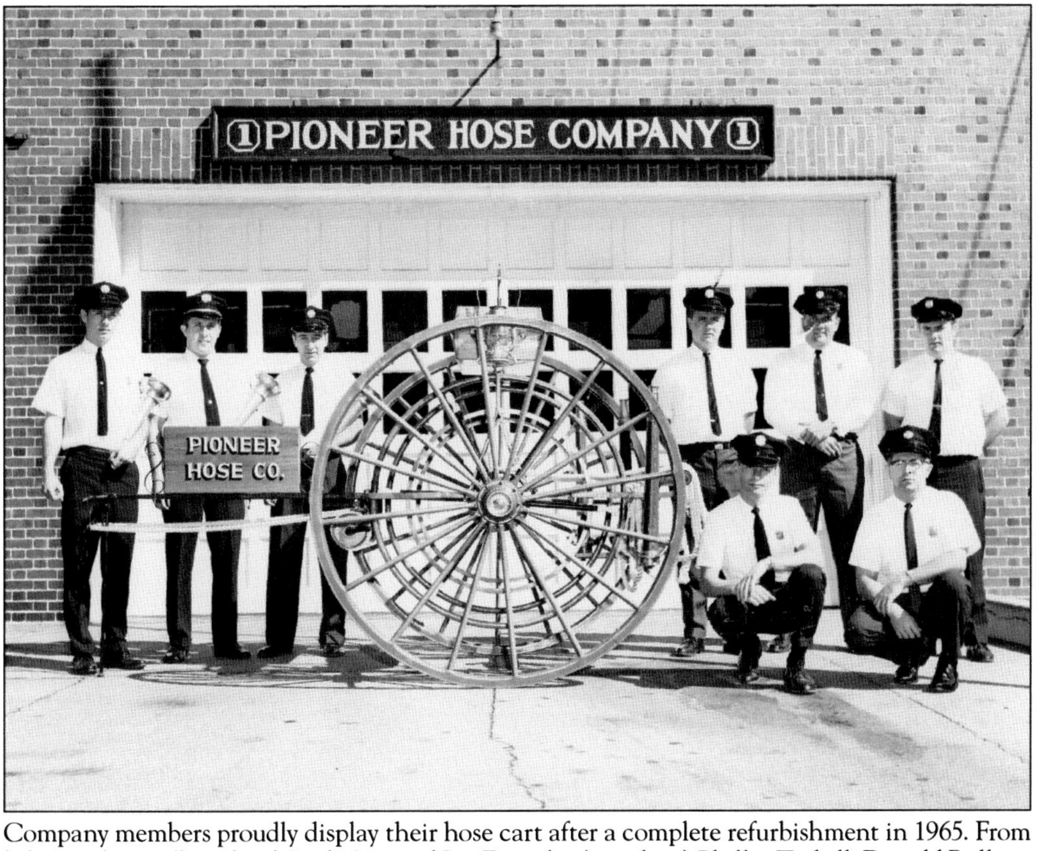

Company members proudly display their hose cart after a complete refurbishment in 1965. From left to right are (kneeling) Dick Gay and Joe Evanski; (standing) Phillip Tuthill, Donald Rollins, Ray Landry, Don McPhail, Jack Lenard, and Alan MacGeachie. (Donald Rollins family.)

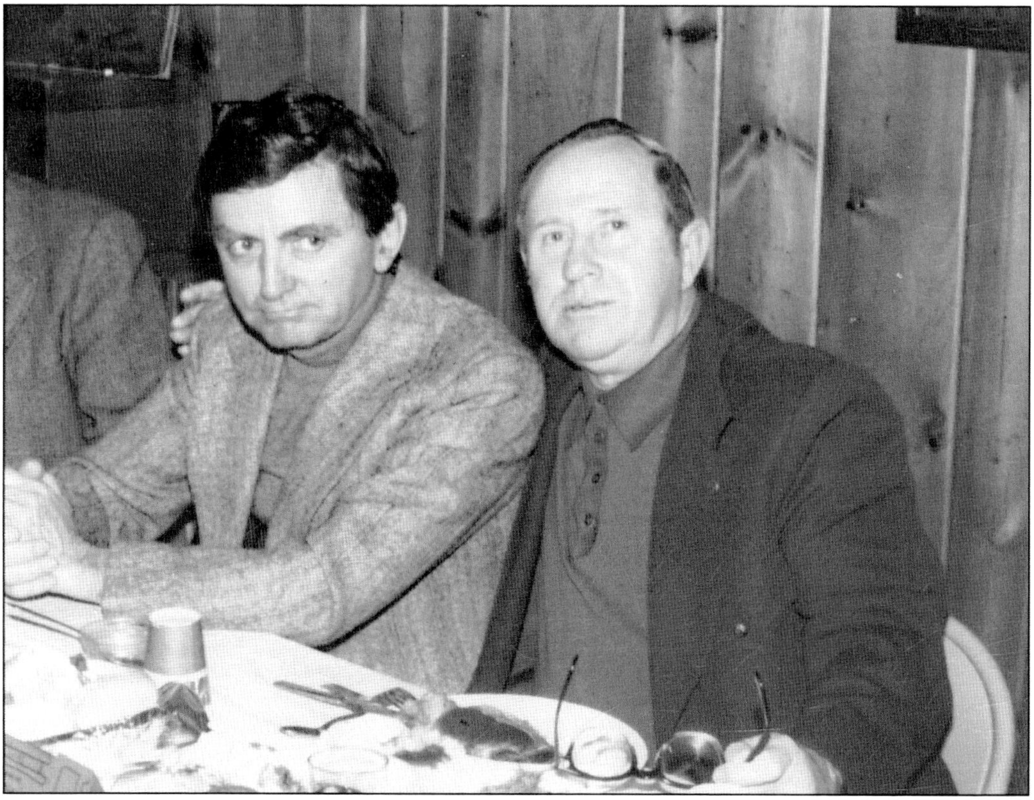

Everest Brustolon (left) and Ray Scully enjoy dinner at an Eastern Point Fire Company banquet in the 1960s. In 2016, the 95-year-old Brustolon was the oldest living member of the fire department's volunteers. (Eastern Point Volunteer Fire Company.)

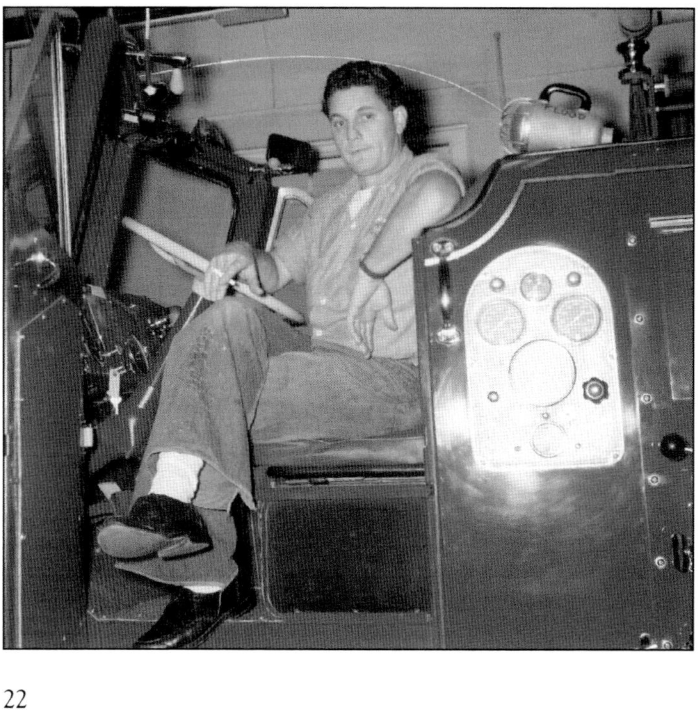

This c. 1960 photograph shows firefighter William Scarano sitting in the 1956 Ward LaFrance. After joining Eastern Point in 1946, Scarano was hired by the Borough of Groton Fire Department in 1954 and was appointed chief in 1968. He held that position until his retirement in 1985. (William Scarano.)

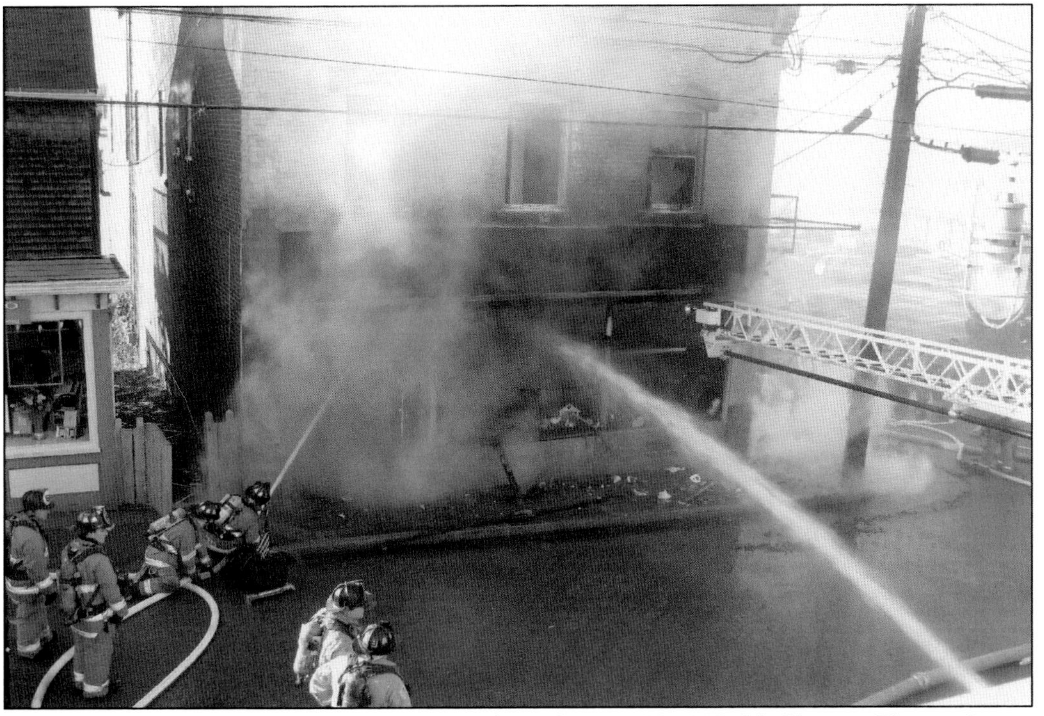

On January 9, 2008, a fast-moving fire grew to three alarms at Ken's Tackle Shop on Thames Street. The building had to be razed, and the business relocated several doors down. (Jim Streeter.)

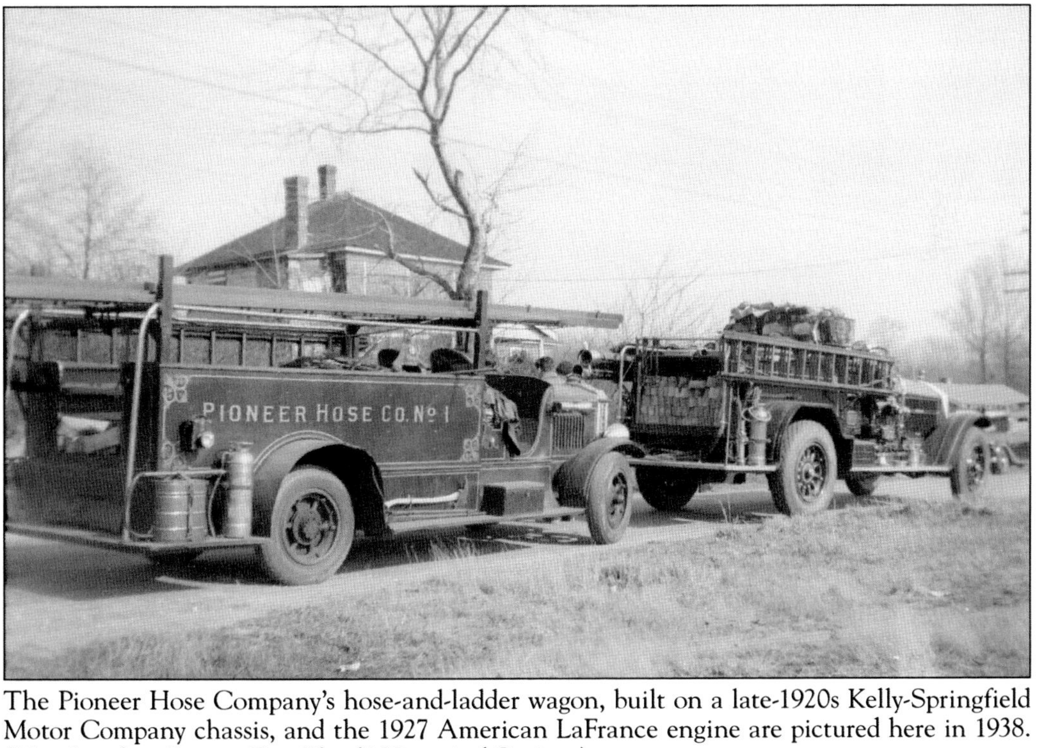

The Pioneer Hose Company's hose-and-ladder wagon, built on a late-1920s Kelly-Springfield Motor Company chassis, and the 1927 American LaFrance engine are pictured here in 1938. (New London County Fire Chiefs' Historical Society.)

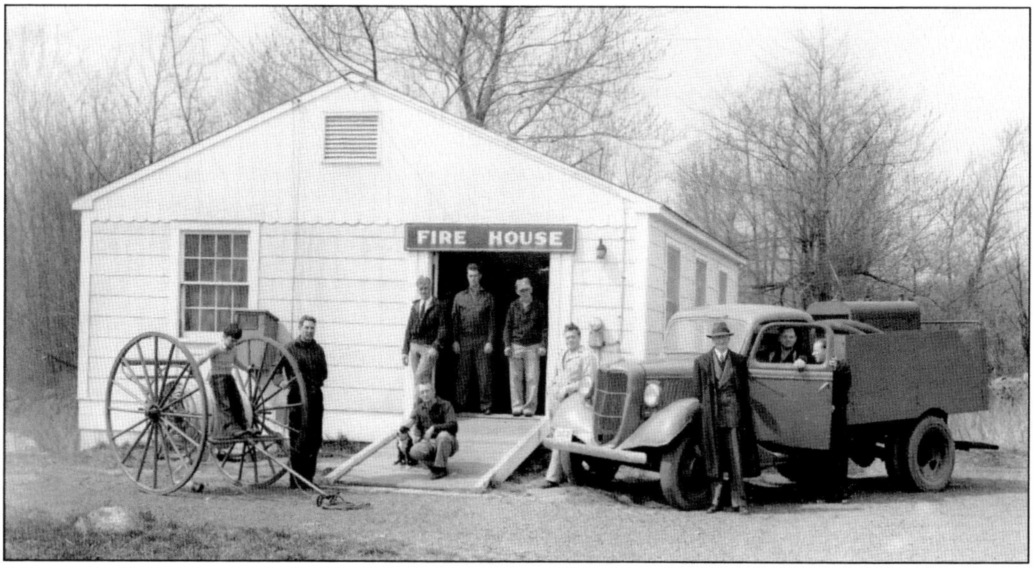

This early-1940s photograph shows volunteers from the Eastern Point Volunteer Fire Company displaying their fire equipment at the Bill Avenue firehouse. (Jim Streeter.)

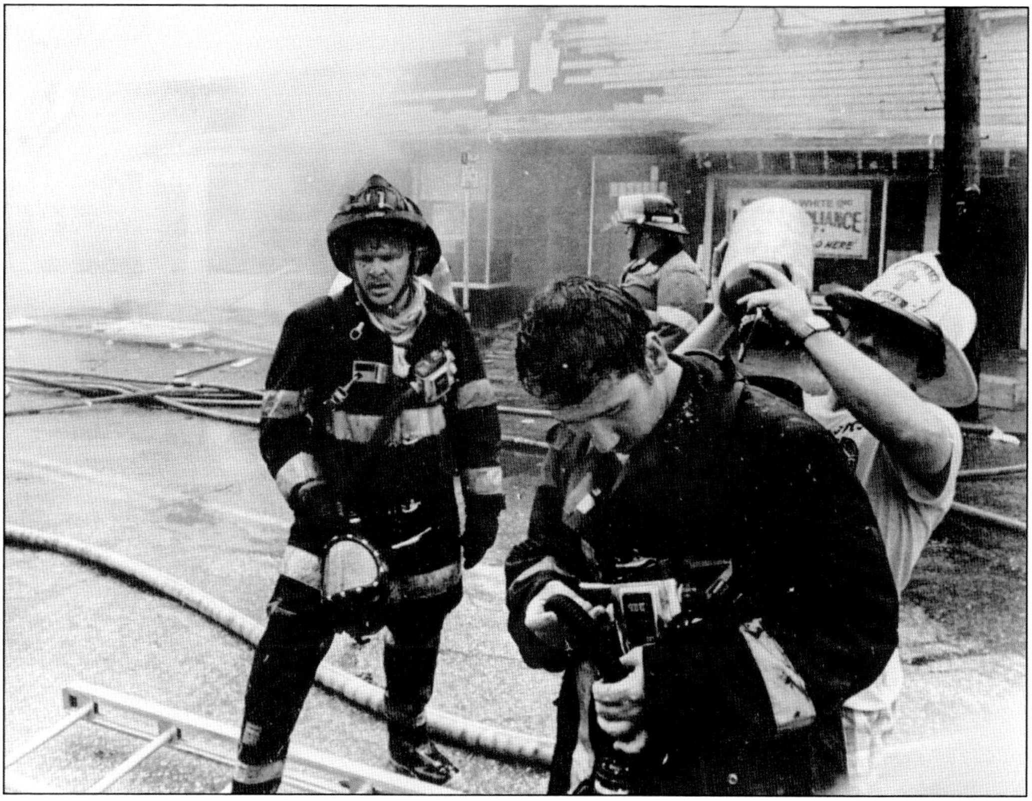

On June 20, 1984, a stubborn fire at the Morgan and White Store on Thames Street caused extensive damage to the building. Pioneer Hose Company member Roger Thayer (left) waits while Eastern Point member Jody DeCarolis has his air bottle changed by chaplain Fr. Larry Ouimett. Pioneer Hose Company member Mike Martin is in the background. (Pioneer Hose Company.)

After a Naval Submarine Base New London fire fought under severe weather conditions in December 1950, Borough of Groton fire chief Herbert White was so impressed with the borough's fire hose that he agreed to endorse it in an advertisement for the hose manufacturer. (Jim Streeter.)

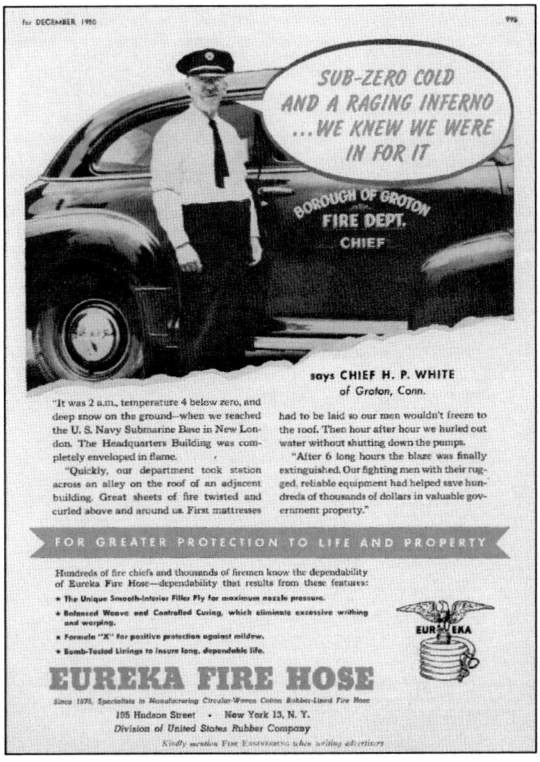

for DECEMBER 1950
SUB-ZERO COLD AND A RAGING INFERNO ...WE KNEW WE WERE IN FOR IT
BOROUGH OF GROTON FIRE DEPT. CHIEF
says CHIEF H. P. WHITE of Groton, Conn.
"It was 2 a.m., temperature 4 below zero, and deep snow on the ground—when we reached the U. S. Navy Submarine Base in New London. The Headquarters Building was completely enveloped in flame.
"Quickly, our department took station across an alley on the roof of an adjacent building. Great sheets of fire twisted and curled above and around us. First mattresses had to be laid so our men wouldn't freeze to the roof. Then hour after hour we hurled out water without shutting down the pumps.
"After 6 long hours the blaze was finally extinguished. Our fighting men with their rugged, reliable equipment had helped save hundreds of thousands of dollars in valuable government property."
FOR GREATER PROTECTION TO LIFE AND PROPERTY
Hundreds of fire chiefs and thousands of firemen know the dependability of Eureka Fire Hose—dependability that results from these features:
★ The Unique Smooth-Interior Filler Ply for maximum nozzle pressure.
★ Balanced Weave and Controlled Curing, which eliminate excessive writhing and warping.
★ Formula "X" for positive protection against mildew.
★ Bomb-Tested Linings to insure long, dependable life.
EUREKA FIRE HOSE
Since 1875, Specialists in Manufacturing Circular-Woven Cotton Rubber-Lined Fire Hose
195 Hudson Street • New York 13, N. Y.
Division of United States Rubber Company

On May 1, 1971, a fire at the El Bolero Bar and Grill caused extensive damage. The morning fire started near the stove and quickly spread when sprinklers in the building failed to operate. (City of Groton Fire Department.)

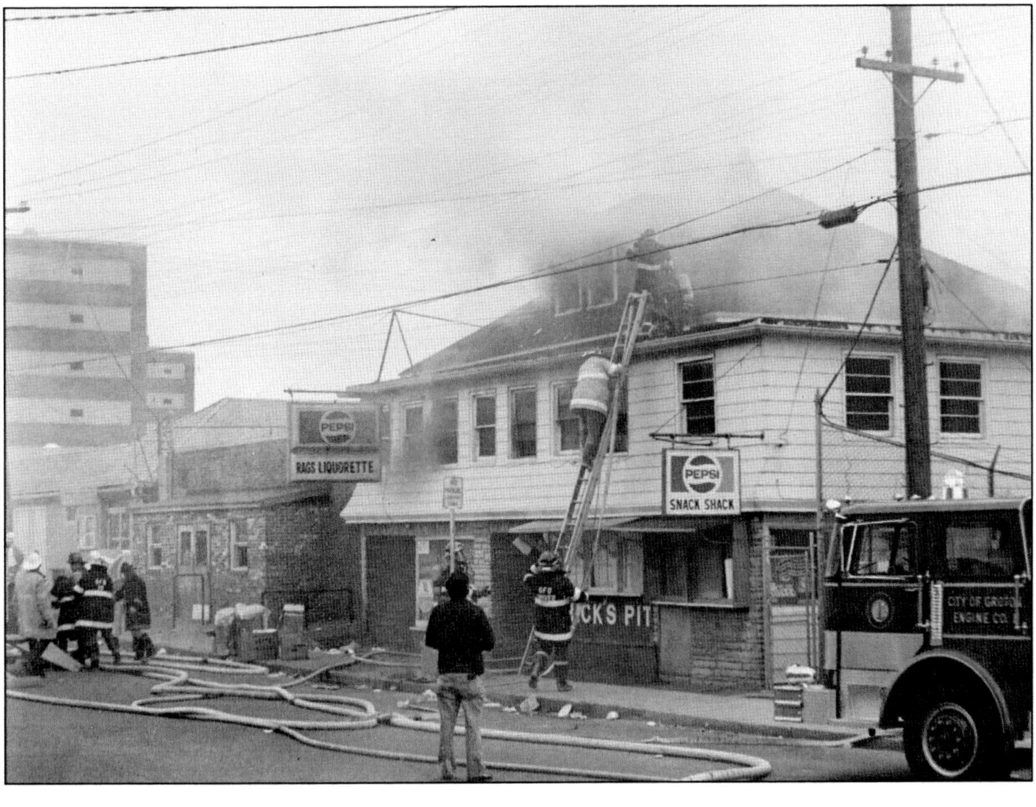

PEPSI
RAGS LIQUORETTE
PEPSI
SNACK SHACK
CITY OF GROTON ENGINE CO.

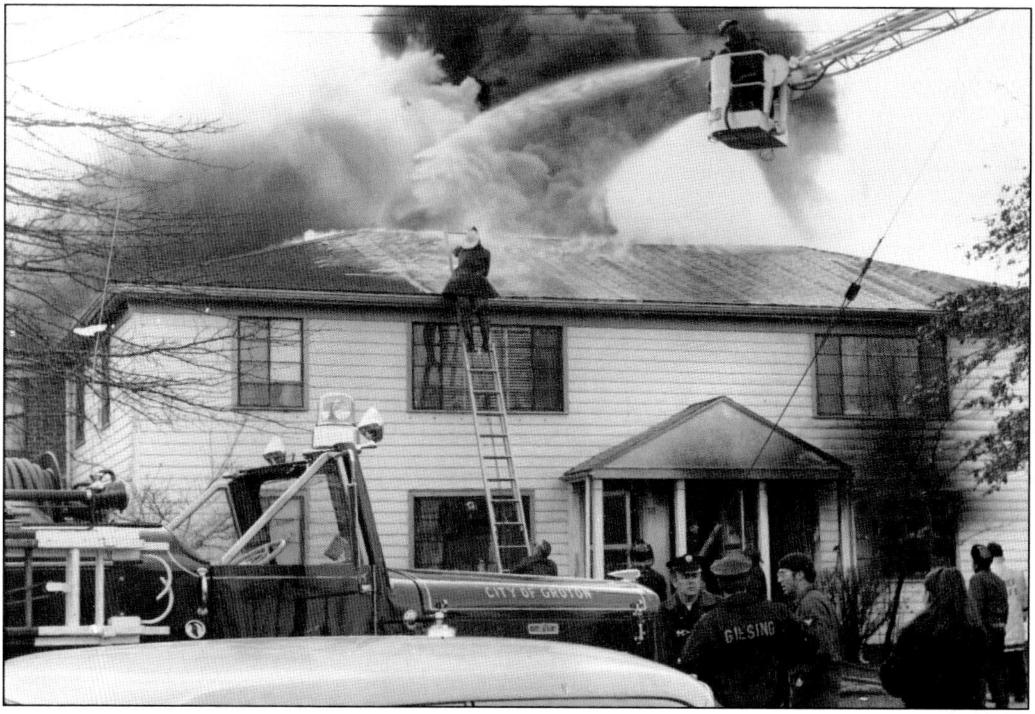

On December 18, 1971, a fire at 19 Bishop Lane heavily damaged the building after a lit candle ignited curtains on a living-room window. The city's three engines, snorkel, and 50 men fought the fire. (Joseph Renda.)

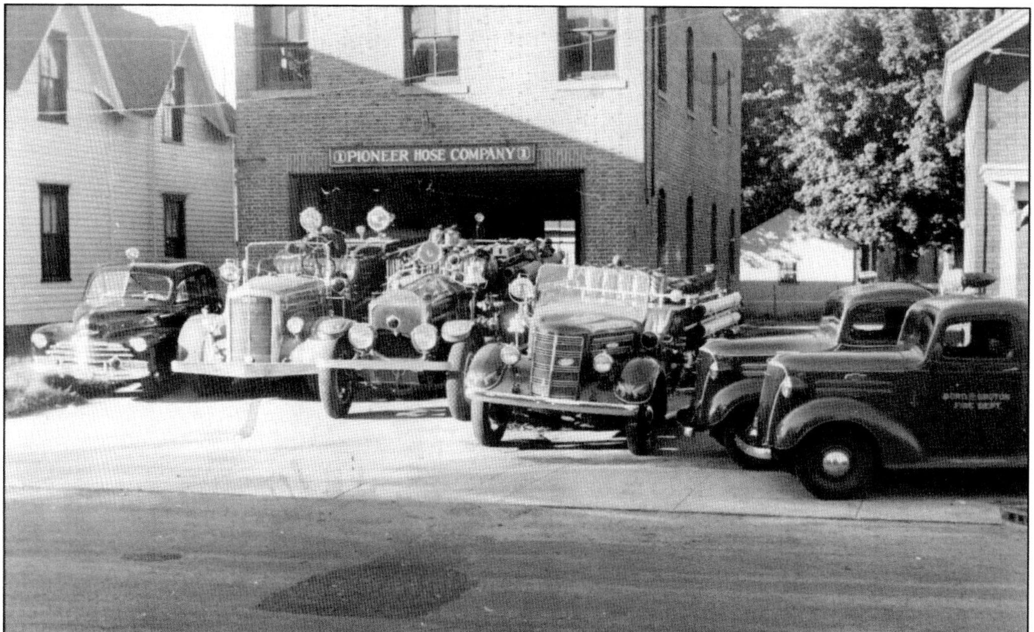

In this 1940s photograph, apparatuses from the Pioneer Hose Company are displayed on the apron. (Jim Streeter.)

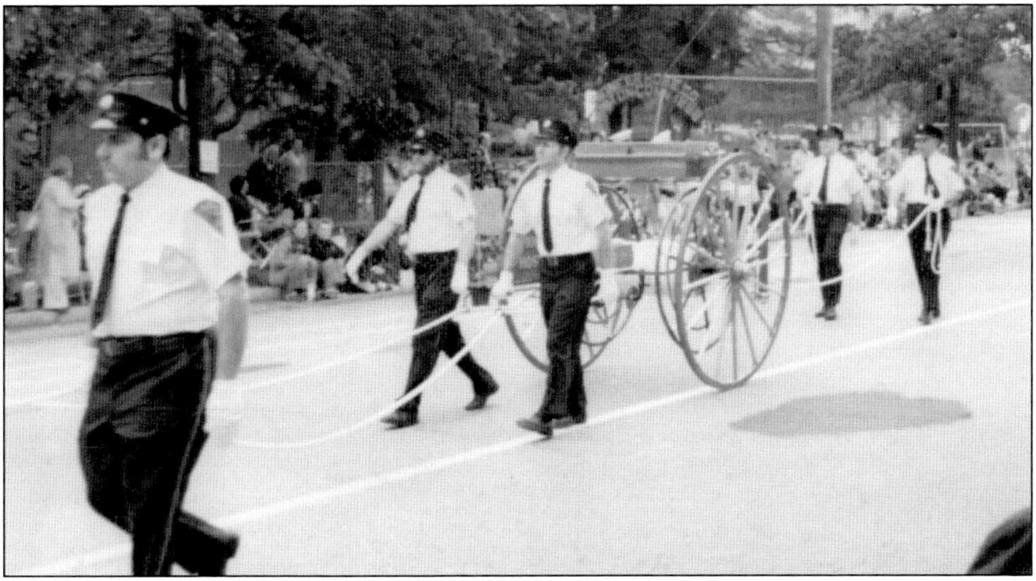

For many years, members of the Pioneer Hose Company proudly led their restored hose reel through parades all over Connecticut, winning many awards. In this c. 1970 image, note the two brakemen with ropes at the rear of the cart; they kept the reel under control while traveling downhill. (Pioneer Hose Company.)

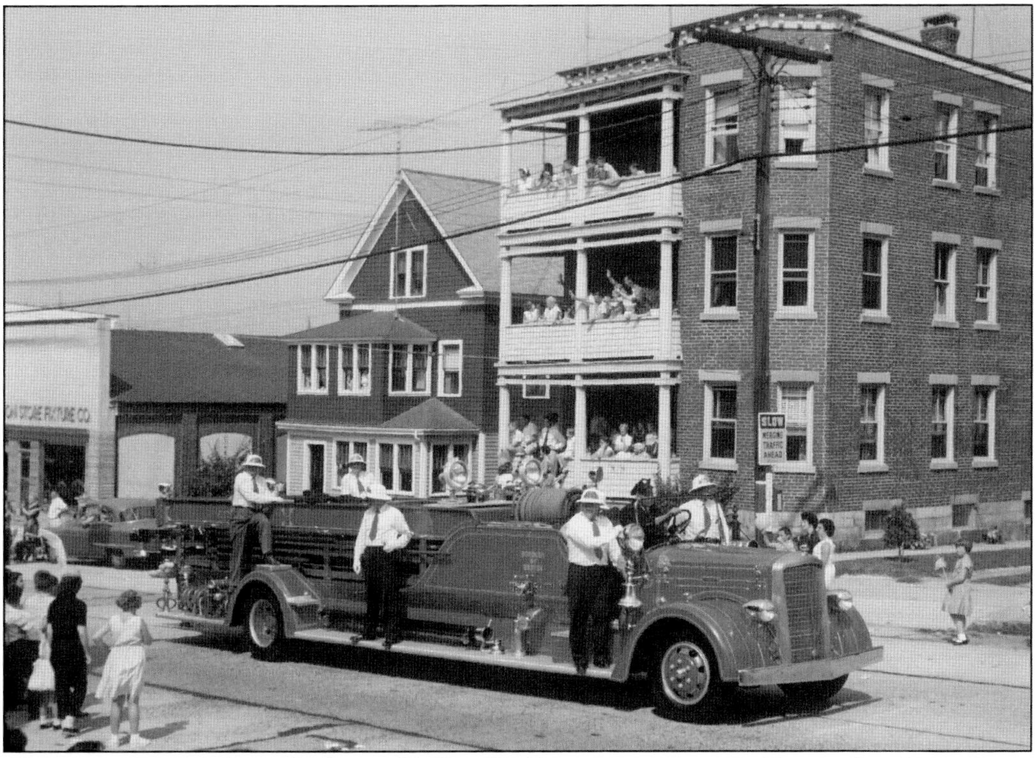

This c. 1966 image shows the borough's Ward LaFrance city service ladder truck making its way down Montauk Avenue on a beautiful day during the State Fireman's Convention parade in New London. The borough purchased the truck for $8,500 in July 1938. (William Scarano.)

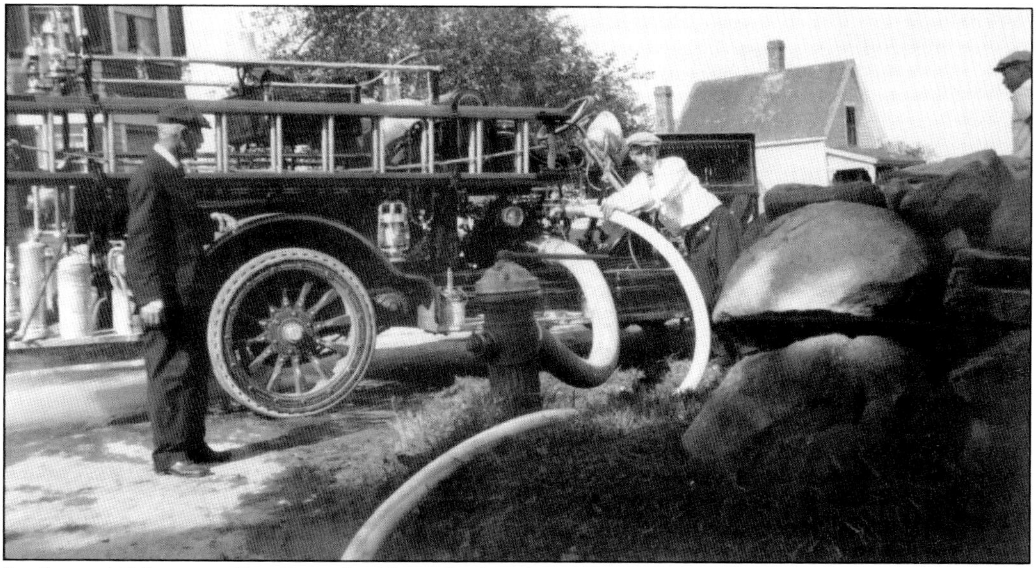

In this c. 1925 image, Ray Fogg (holding the hose) operates the 1917 American LaFrance engine from a hydrant as George Hempstead (at left) watches. This engine was used until 1932, when the Pioneer Hose Company gave it to the Boston & Maine Railroad. (Jim Streeter.)

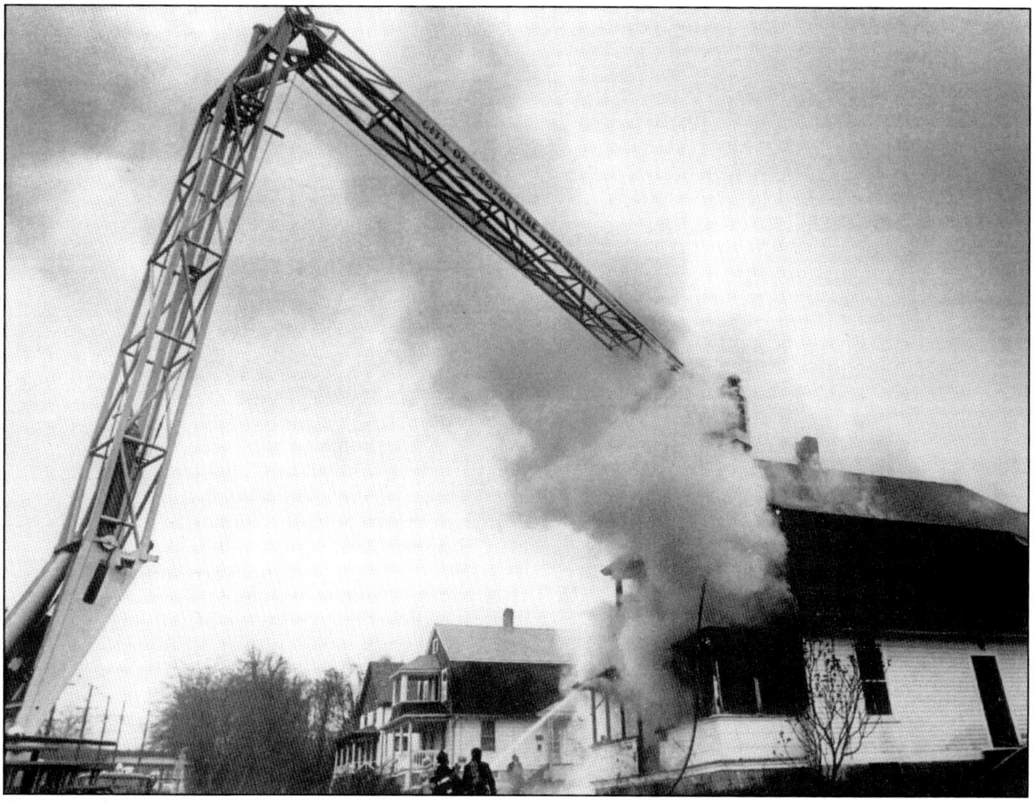

On March 17, 1982, a fire started at 368 Poquonnock Road when a quartz heater ignited a bed in the first-floor apartment. A Bridge Street Auto Company worker noticed the billowing smoke and reported the fire. (City of Groton Fire Department.)

The Mystic Bridge Fire Engine Company, which was established in 1846, was the first organized fire company in Mystic. This company was in existence for only a few years. In 1874, the Mezeppa Fire Company was formed and was located on Holmes Street. In July 1875, the B.F. Hoxie Engine Company was formed, and the Mystic Fire District was created four years later. (Mystic Fire Department.)

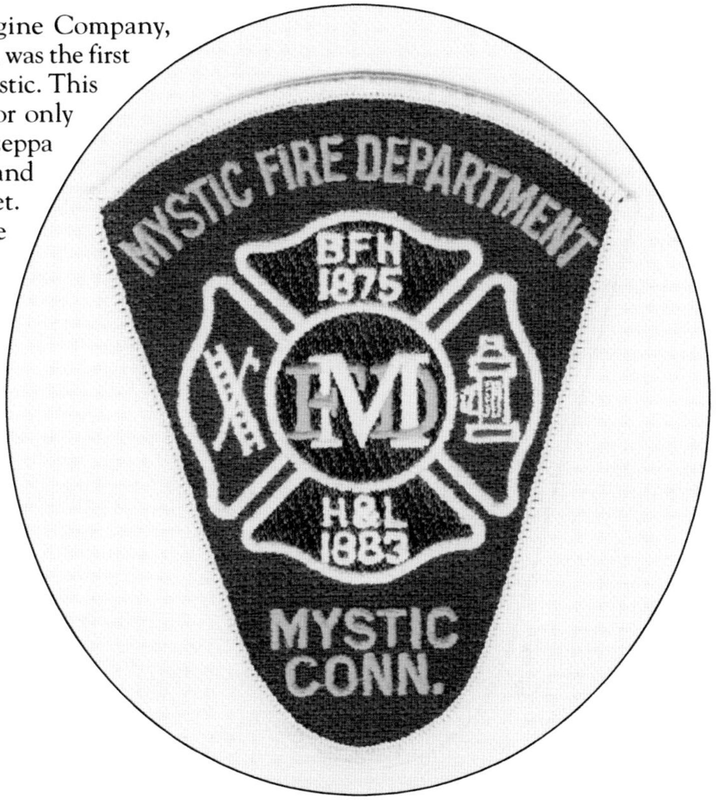

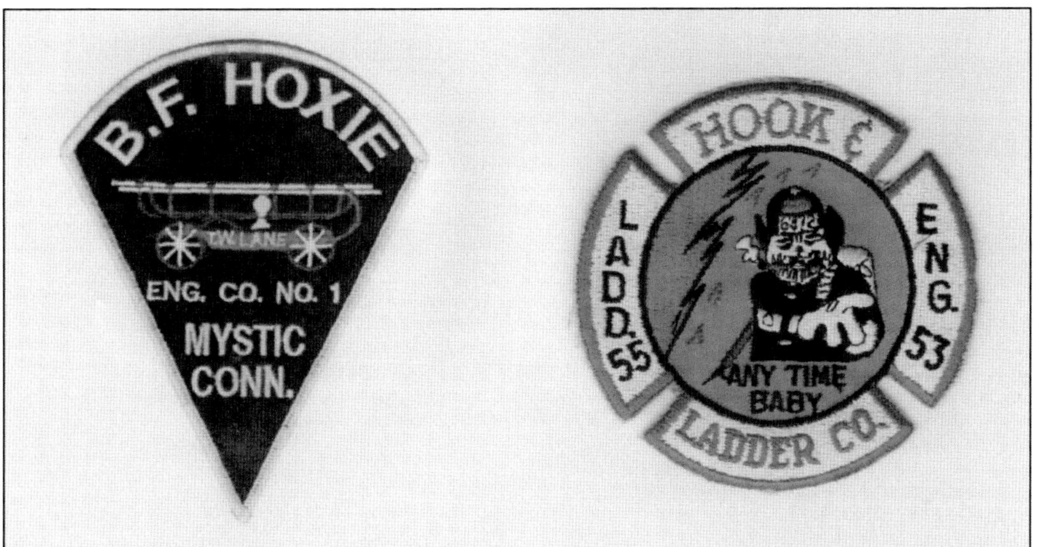

In 1875, after the Oceanic Woolen Mill Fire, Benjamin F. Hoxie donated $1,000 toward the purchase of a Hunneman and Company steam fire engine. His donation spurred others and made the purchase possible. After the engine was delivered, the steamer and the company were named after Hoxie. In 1883, Mystic Hook and Ladder Company was formed; the new fire company moved into their own quarters on Gravel Street in 1884 and relocated to their current location on New London Road in 1967. (Mystic Fire Department.)

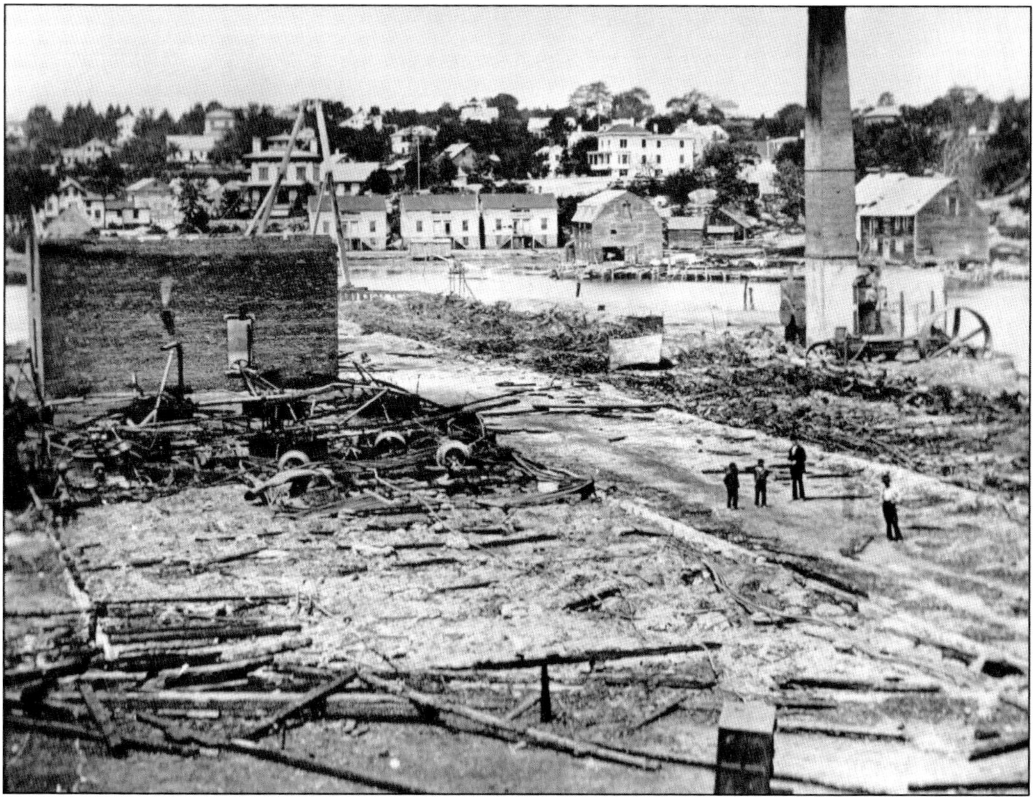

The 1875 fire at the Oceanic Woolen Mill and the Mystic Iron Works was probably the most spectacular fire in the history of Mystic. Lost in the conflagration were a foundry, a blacksmith shop, and two large storehouses. (Mystic Fire Department.)

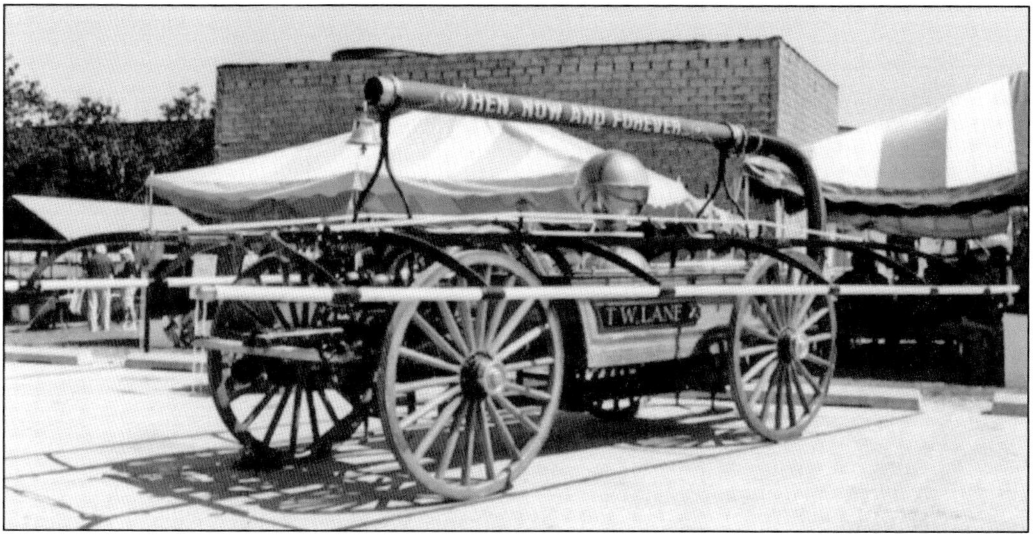

This 1883 Button and Son hand pumper with serial number 688 was built for Greenville, South Carolina. After being acquired in New Hampshire in 1903 for use in musters, it changed hands several times before being purchased by the Hoxie Company in 1967. They have used it for muster competitions ever since. (Mystic Fire Department.)

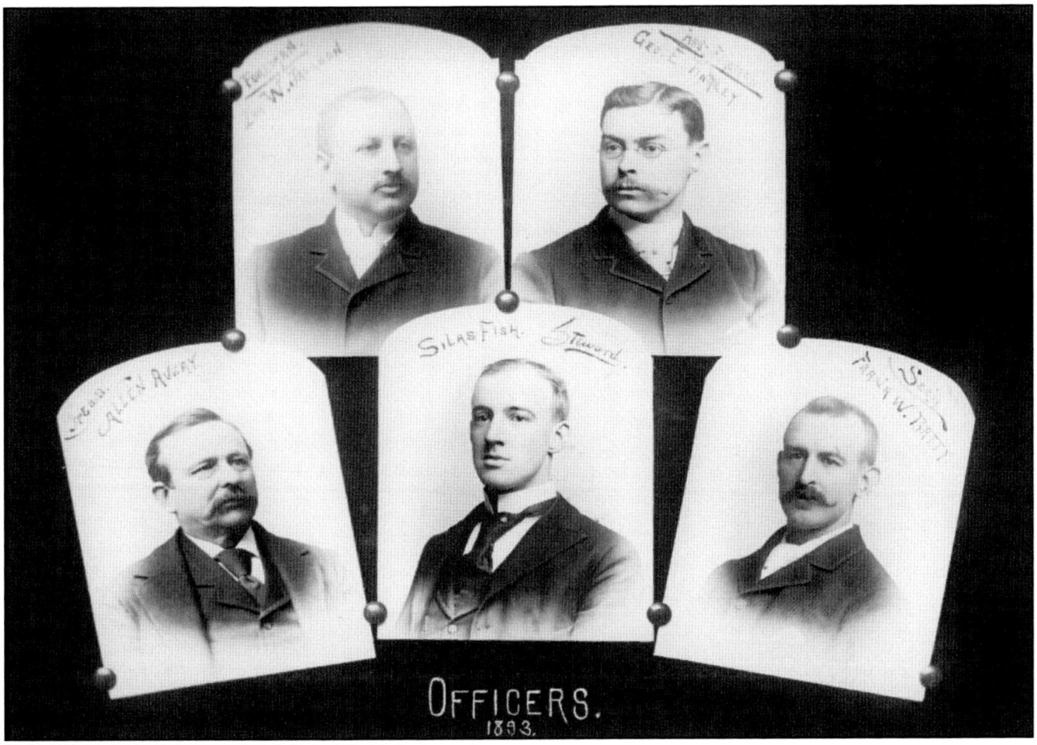

The officers of the Mystic Hook and Ladder Company are pictured here in 1892. Ira Jackson (upper left) and Allen Avery (lower left) were charter officers, and Frank W. Batty (lower right) was a charter member. (Mystic Fire Department.)

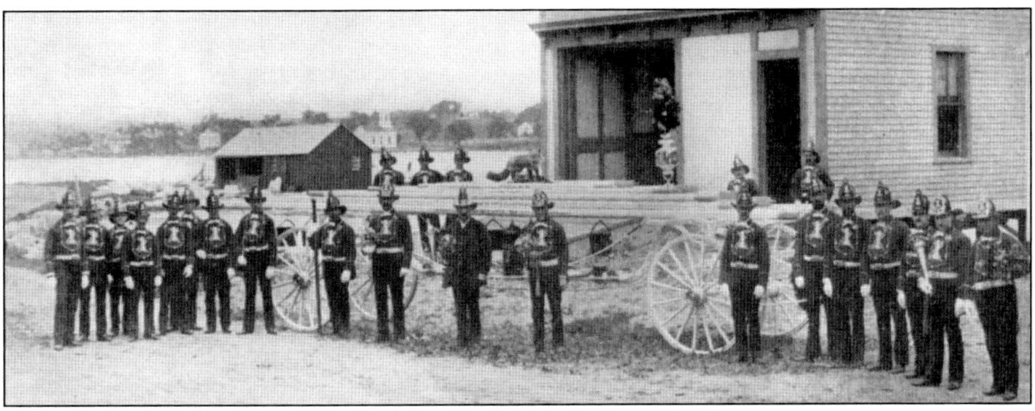

Members of the Mystic Hook and Ladder Company pose with their first apparatus on July 4, 1883. The $380 truck was often referred to as a "lily" due to its numerous coats of white paint. The company eventually sold it to Leominster, Massachusetts, for $450. (Mystic Fire Department.)

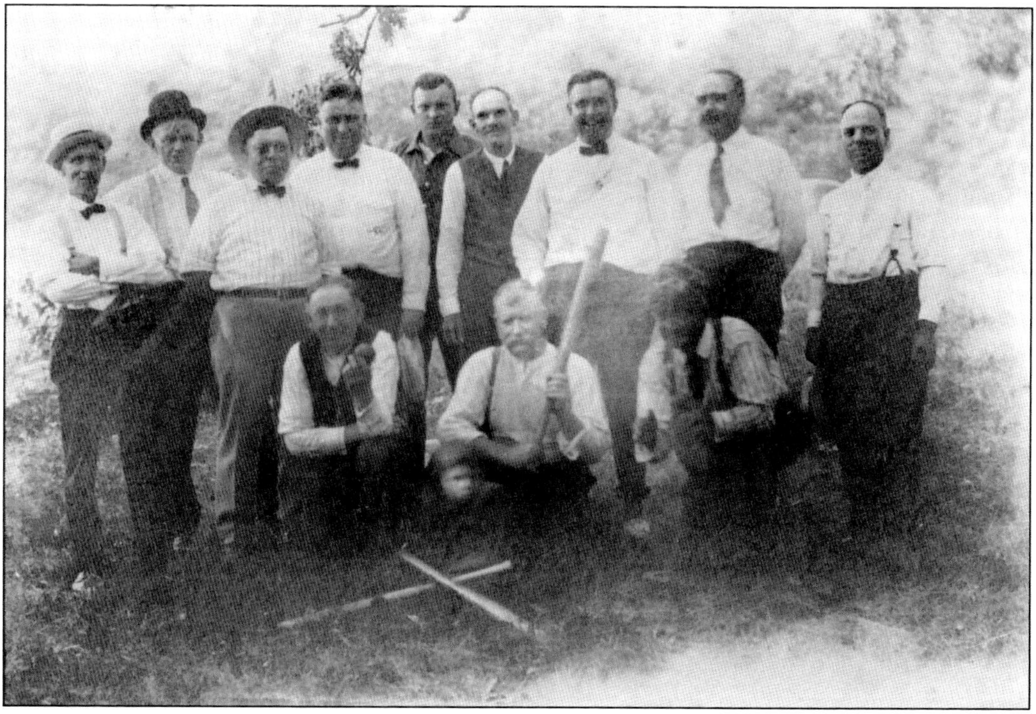

Pictured here around 1900 is the B.F. Hoxie baseball team. From left to right are (kneeling) Charles Foley, Sam Stewart Sr., and Walt Sheehan Sr.; (standing) Chris Rattigan, Jim Foley, Manual Sylvia, George Costello, Frank Goodwin, Bob O'Neil, Connie Costello, ? Donahue Sr., and Jim Fribbauce. (Mystic Fire Department.)

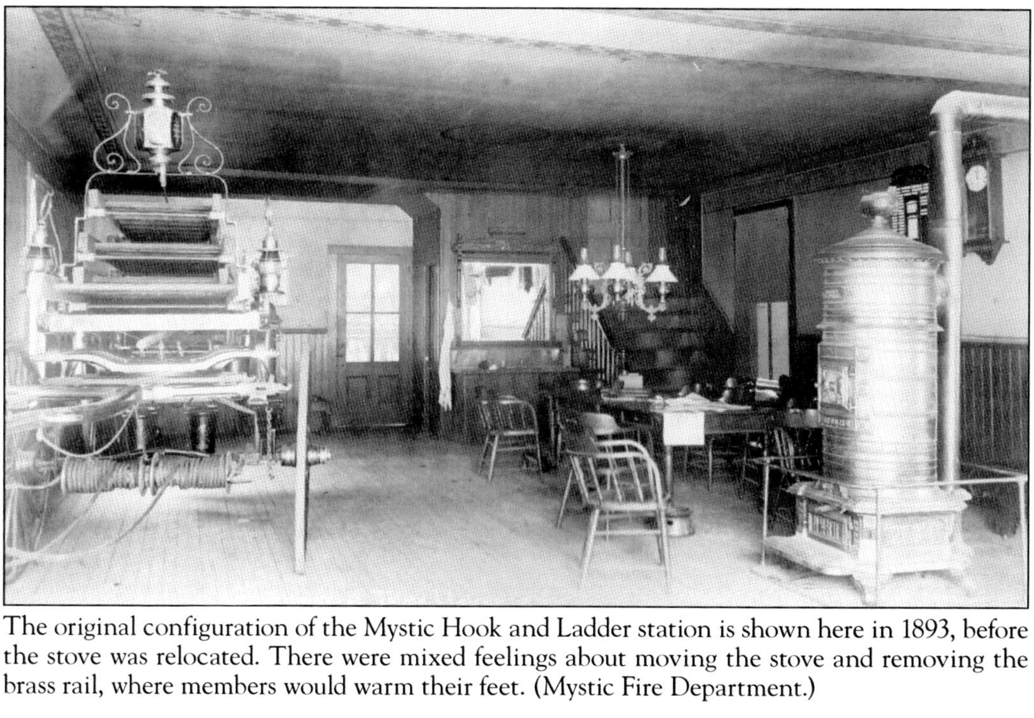

The original configuration of the Mystic Hook and Ladder station is shown here in 1893, before the stove was relocated. There were mixed feelings about moving the stove and removing the brass rail, where members would warm their feet. (Mystic Fire Department.)

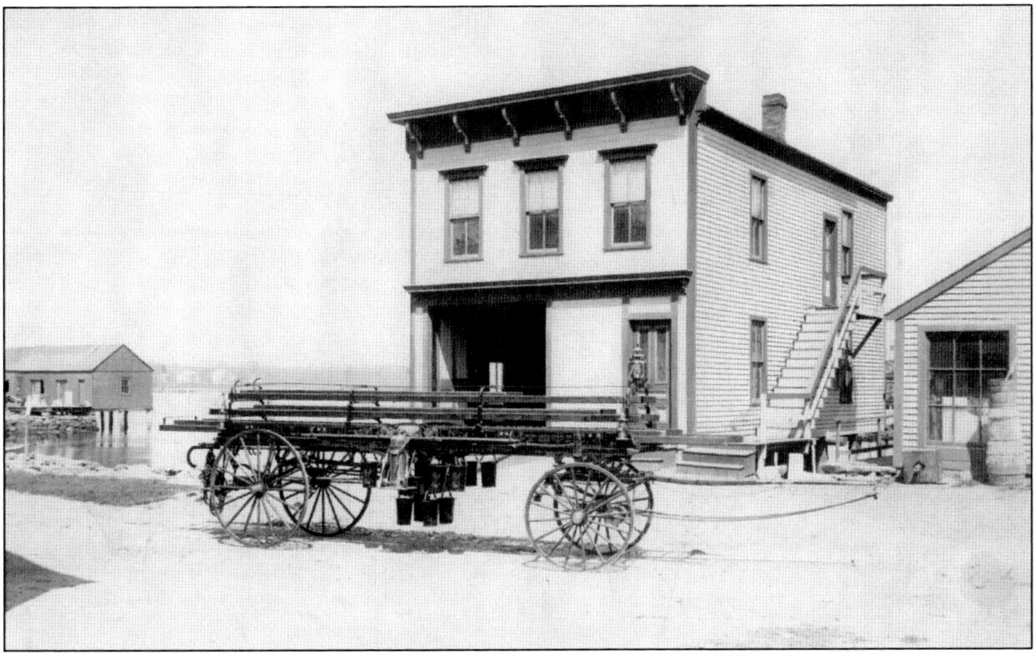

The Mystic Hook and Ladder Company's second apparatus sits outside the Gravel Street quarters in this c. 1890 photograph. It was purchased on December 6, 1887, for $635 and remained in service until 1918. (Mystic Fire Department.)

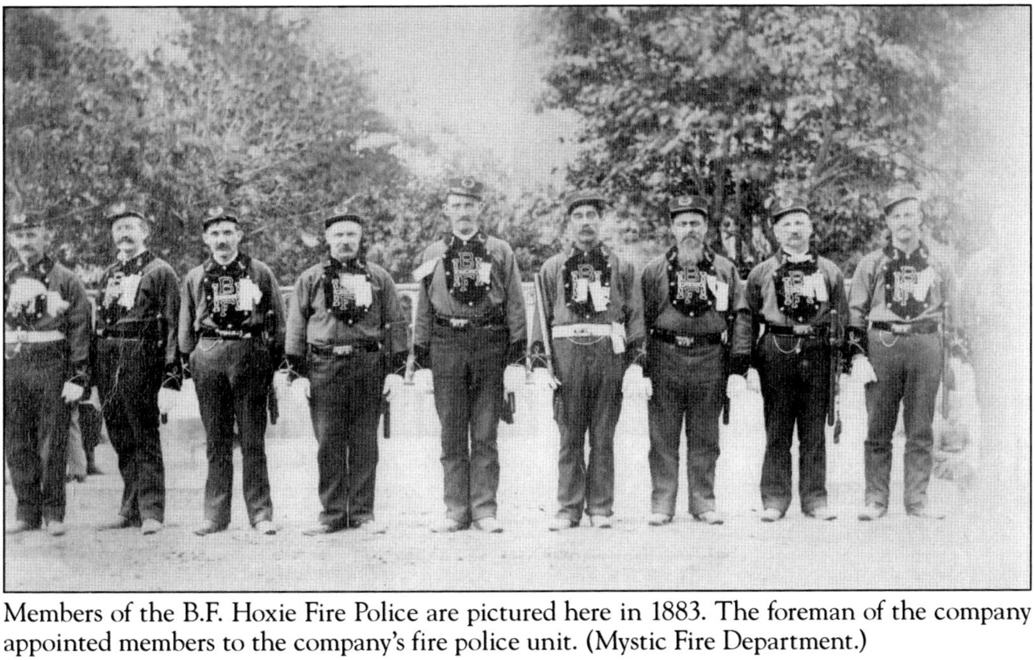

Members of the B.F. Hoxie Fire Police are pictured here in 1883. The foreman of the company appointed members to the company's fire police unit. (Mystic Fire Department.)

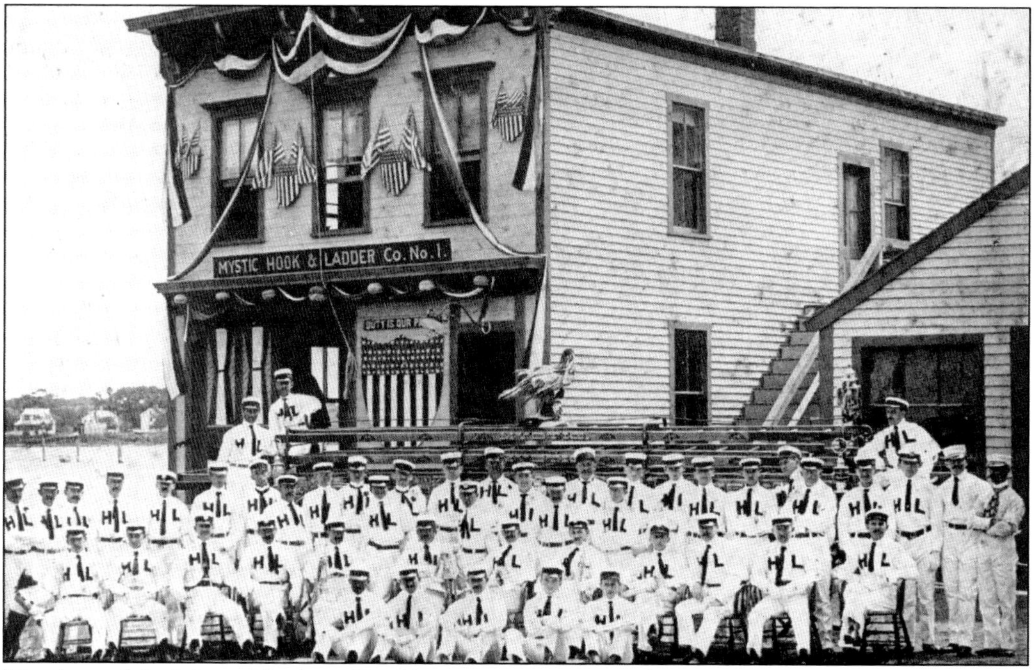

Members of the Mystic Hook and Ladder Company pose with their ladder truck in front of their company headquarters on July 4, 1901, before the annual Fourth of July parade. In 1884, the company paid $200 to purchase the property upon which this building sits. Construction costs for the building totaled $1,100. (Mystic Fire Department.)

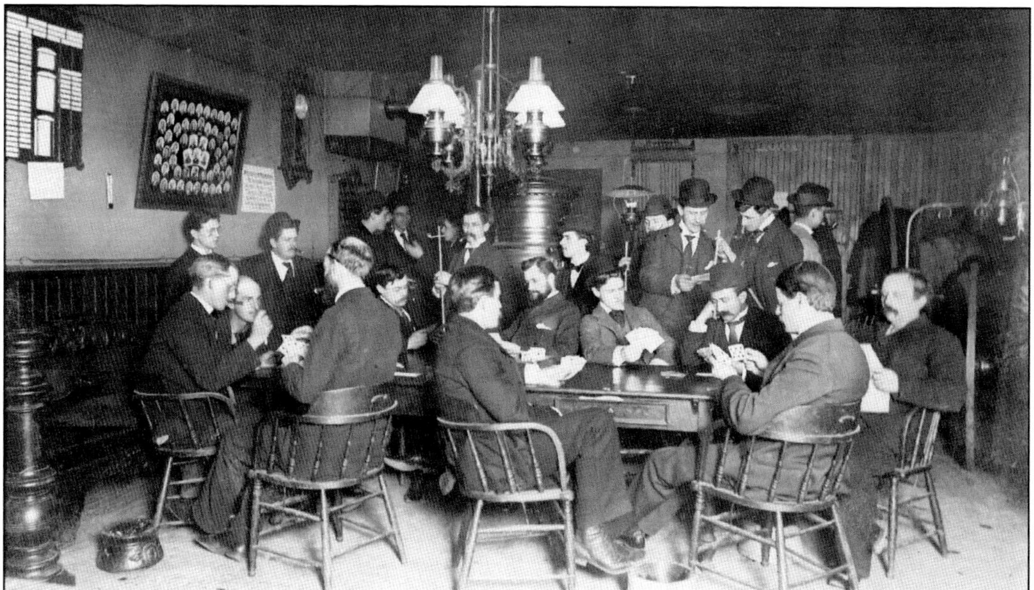

In the 1880s, fire companies were hubs of social activity; card games and pool and darts tournaments were frequent events. While looking at this c. 1895 image, note the framed photographs of charter members on the wall at left; the company still proudly displays this in their current company quarters. The spittoons were replaced with ash receivers in 1940. (Mystic Fire Department.)

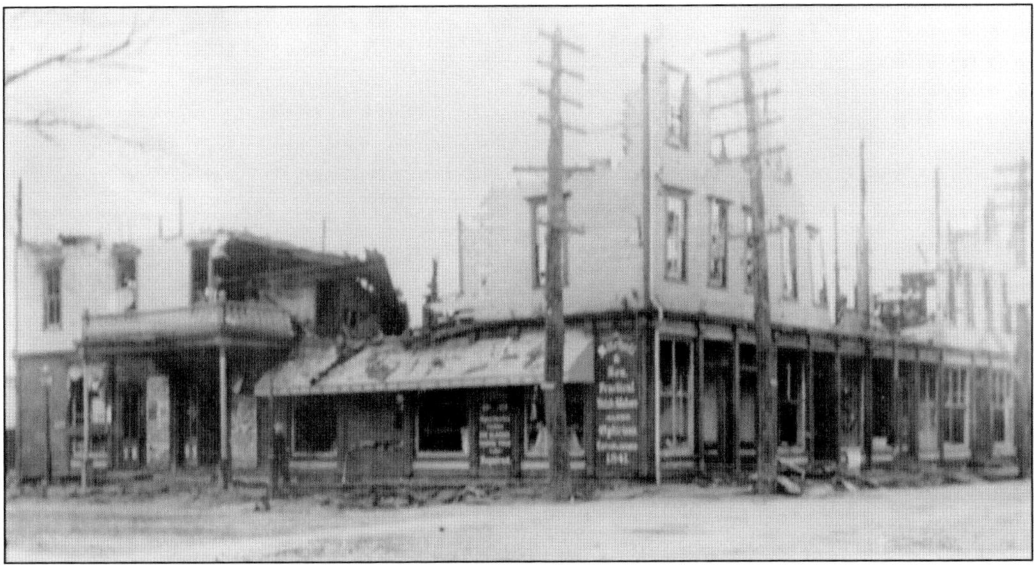

This photograph shows damage to the Mystic Opera House after a fire in November 1900. Both Mystic companies responded, and the services of the Stonington Steamers Engine Company were also required. Although the opera house was a total loss, the fire was kept from adjoining structures. (Mystic Fire Department.)

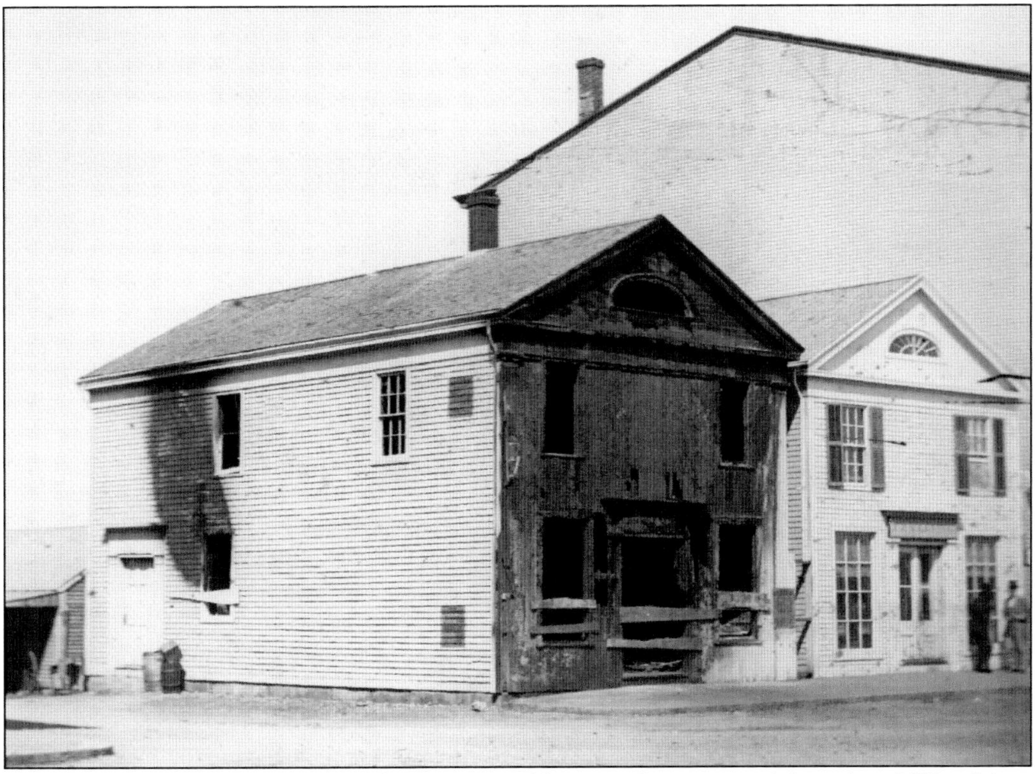

In April 1877, a fire broke out in the Evans Building on the corner of Gravel and West Main Streets. The B.F. Hoxie Company's new steamer promptly arrived on the scene and put two hose streams on the fire, quickly extinguishing it. (Mystic Fire Department.)

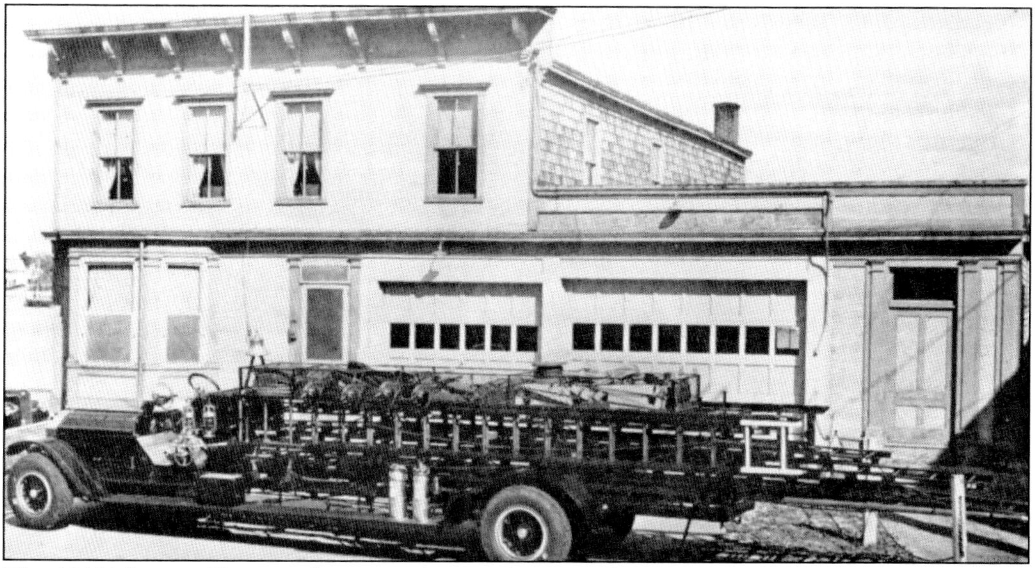

The 1915 Thomas Flyer truck, pictured around 1916, ushered in the motorized era. When the hose bed was full—and with several men standing on the rear step—the front wheels would lift off the ground. This flaw stemmed from improper design by the Providence, Rhode Island, manufacturer. In 1923, the Flyer chassis was replaced with a Sanford chassis, which was nearly (if not just) as unsatisfactory. (Mystic Fire Department.)

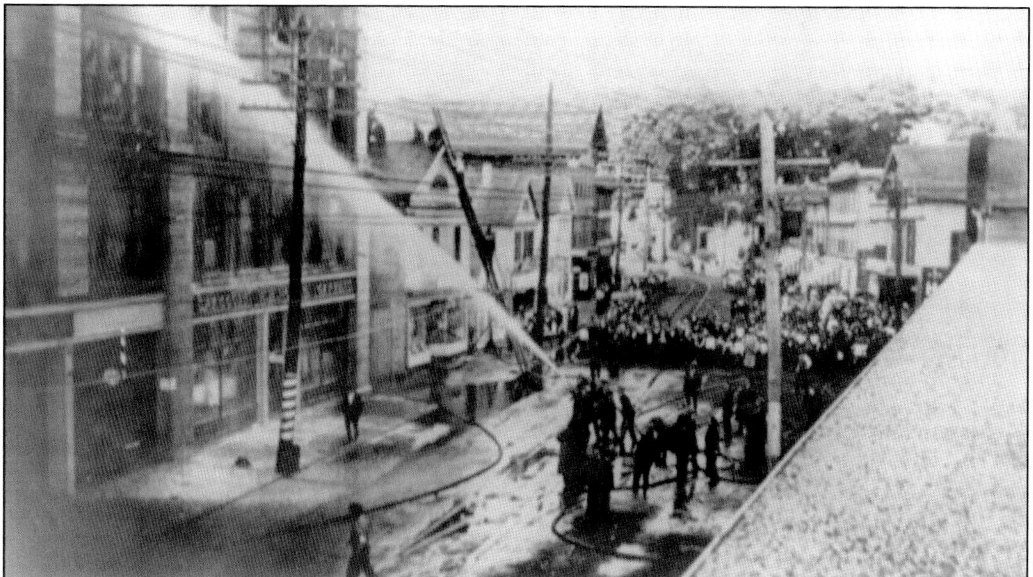

This 1915 fire in the six-year-old Gilbert Block started in the scenery of a theater on the third floor. Since Mystic firefighters did not have a mechanical fire apparatus, they were assisted by the Niagara Hose Company of New London and the Noank Hose Company. (Mystic Fire Department.)

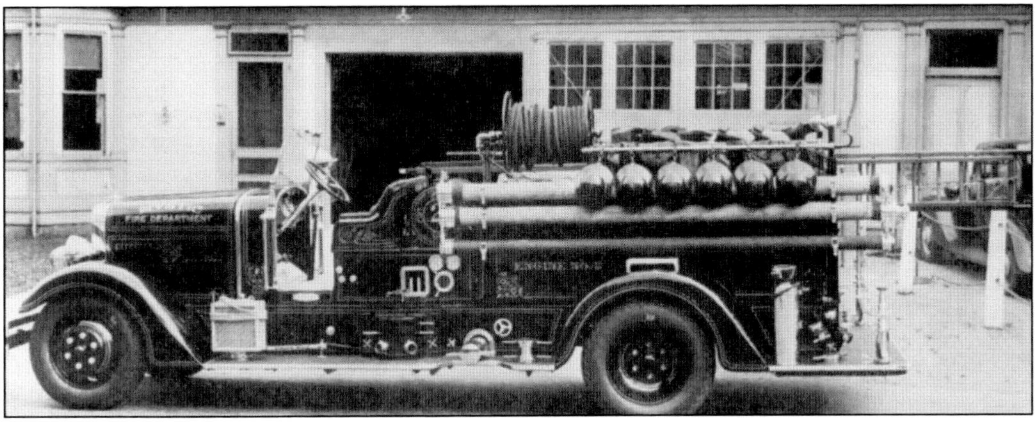

Pictured here around 1936 is the Mystic Hook and Ladder Company's 1936 Seagrave 500-gallon-per-minute engine. It replaced the Sanford ladder truck and remained in service until 1957. (Mystic Fire Department.)

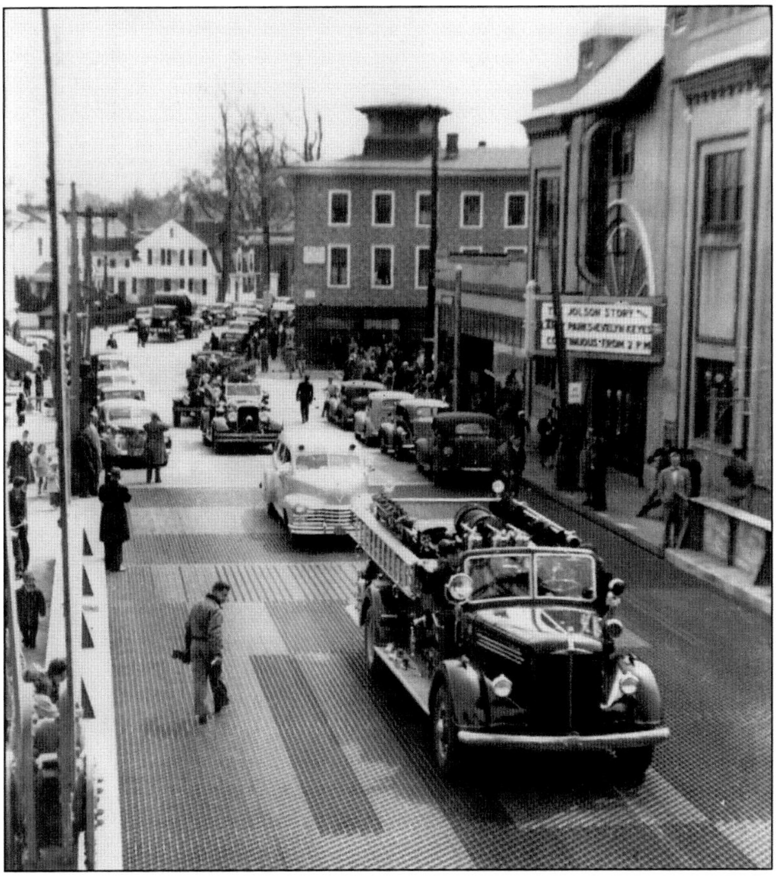

This photograph from May 1947 shows the new Hoxie Mack engine and the new Hoxie Cadillac ambulance. The parade was to support the Fitch Band Boosters Club. Sam Brustolon (holding a camera) is walking on the bridge near the engine, and Bill Dodge, owner of the Cottrell Lumber Company, is standing at the end of the bridge beam at right. (Mystic Fire Department.)

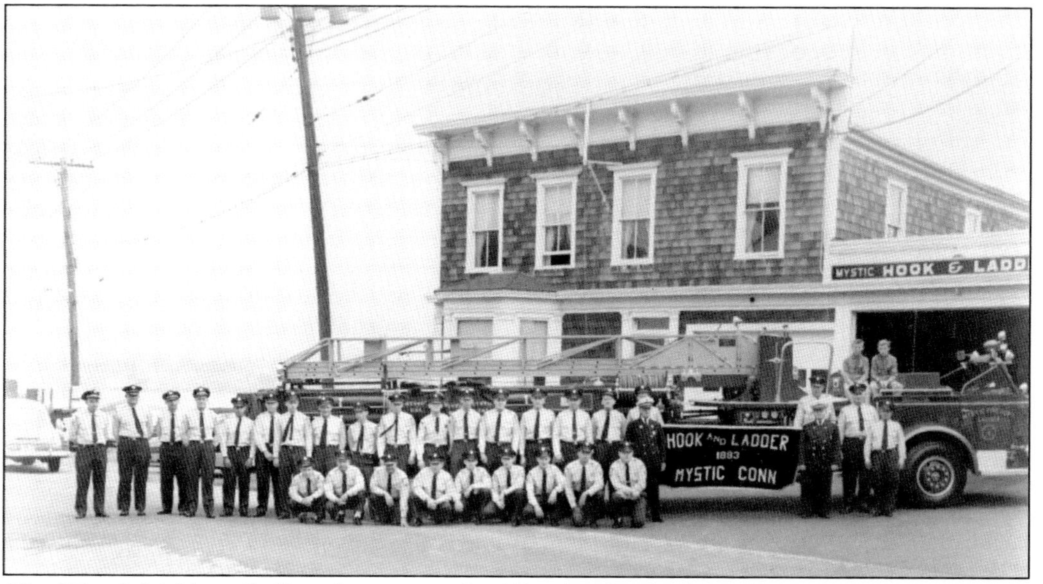

Chief Frank Mabbett (left) and assistant chief Frank Clay, both in dress coats and white hats flanking the banner, pose with members of the Mystic Hook and Ladder Company and their American LaFrance ladder truck, purchased for $35,000 in 1957. This late-1950s photograph was taken in front of their Gravel Street quarters. (Mystic Fire Department.)

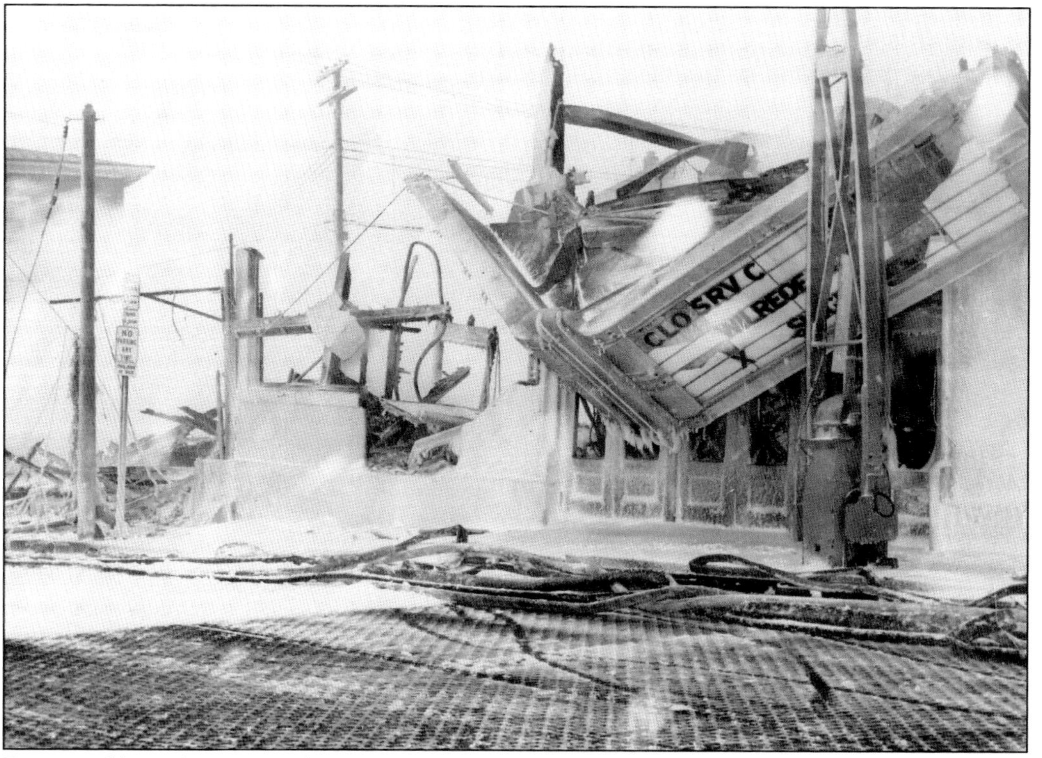

During a blizzard on December 12, 1960, a major fire broke out on the Stonington side of the Mystic River Bridge. The fire destroyed more than a dozen buildings and caused over $1 million in damage. (Mystic Fire Department.)

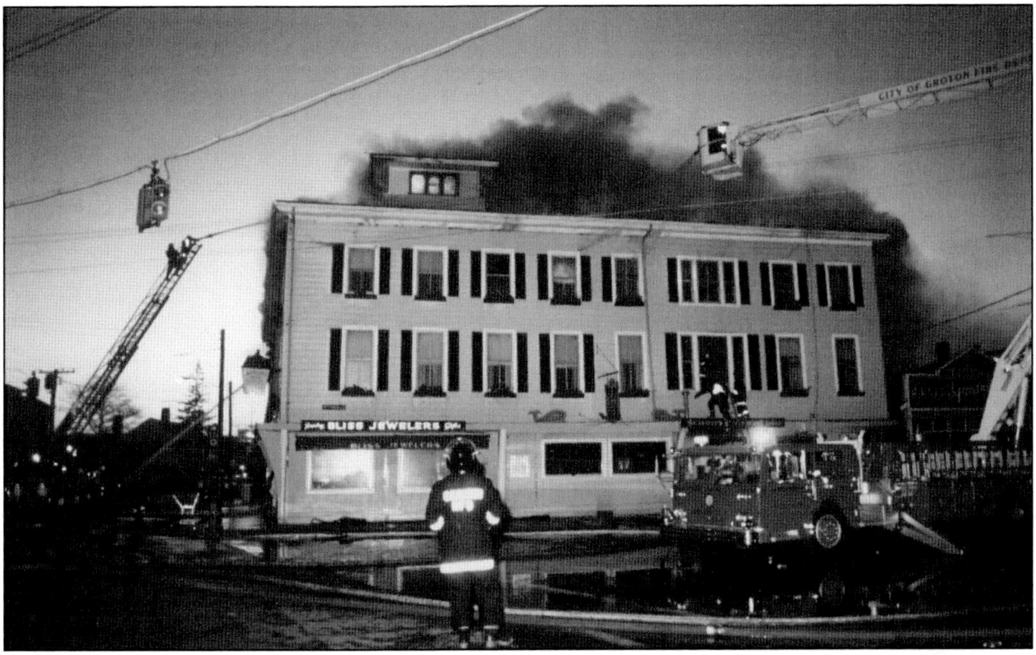

On January 2, 1975, fire struck the Whaler's Inn at 20 East Main Street. The hotel, which opened one month before the start of the Civil War, was heavily damaged. The fire, which started in the kitchen of the Seaport Restaurant, took eight fire companies five hours to extinguish. (Mystic Fire Department.)

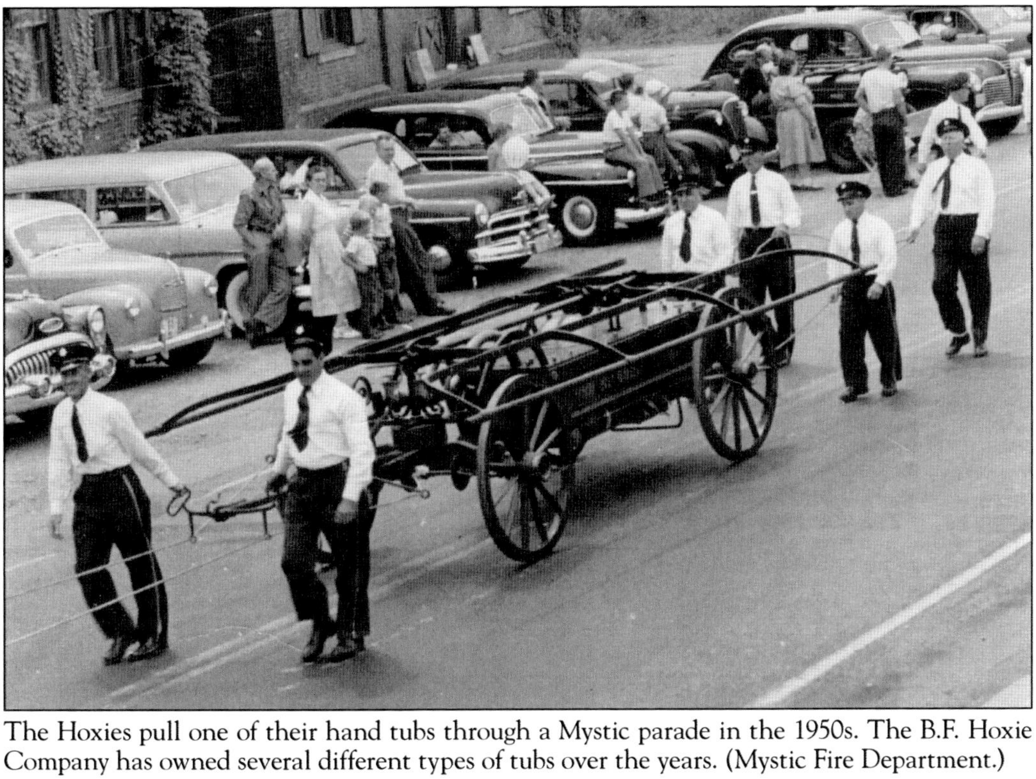

The Hoxies pull one of their hand tubs through a Mystic parade in the 1950s. The B.F. Hoxie Company has owned several different types of tubs over the years. (Mystic Fire Department.)

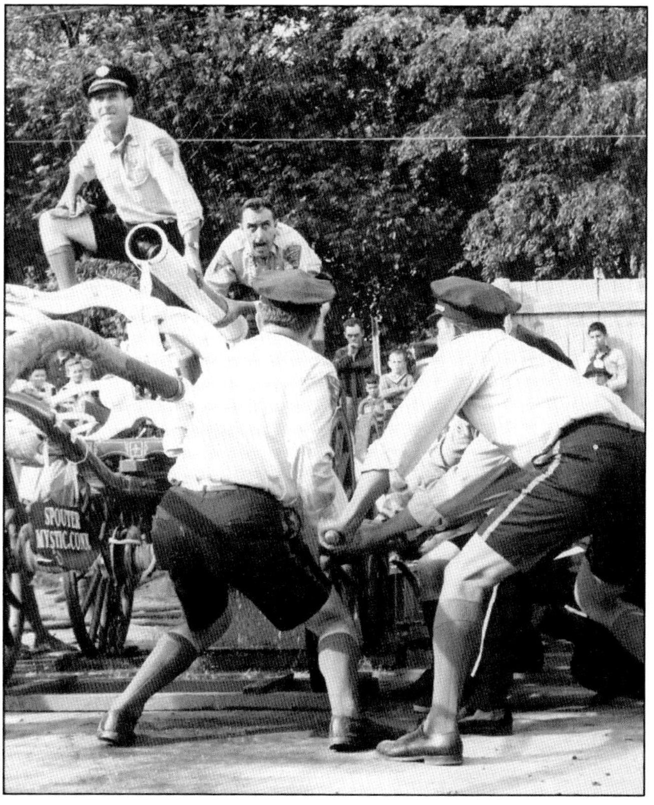

Members of the Hoxie Company pump their hand tub at the Rhode Island state muster in Westerly, Rhode Island, on September 15, 1963. The two foremen on top of the pumper—Albert Brooks (left) and Bob Hartley—are ensuring a good stream is maintained. (Mystic Fire Department.)

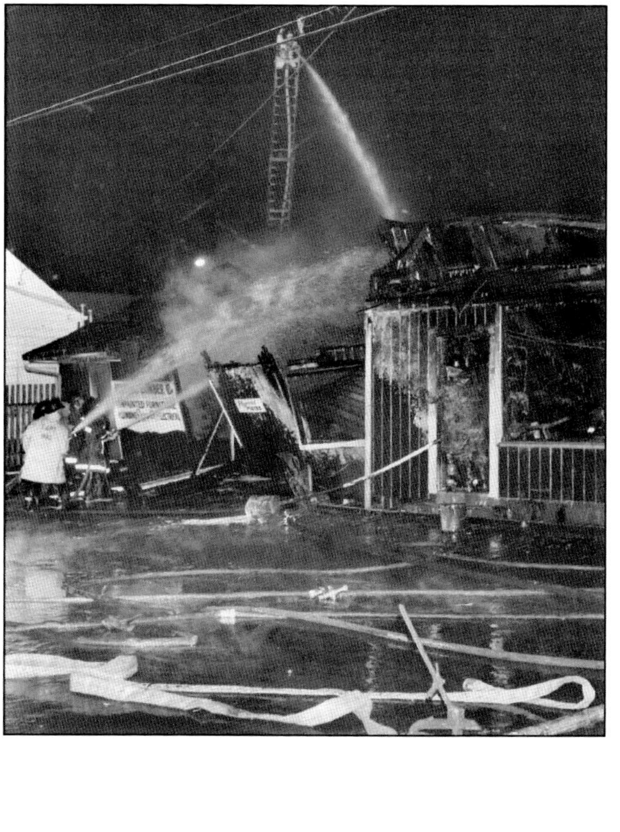

On January 9, 1966, a Mystic fireman was passing by the Mystic Lumber Company on Washington Street when he noticed a fire and pulled the alarm. Six area fire departments were called in to stop the blaze from spreading to the Broadway Avenue Sunoco station only 10 feet away; they were successful in their endeavors. (Mystic Fire Department.)

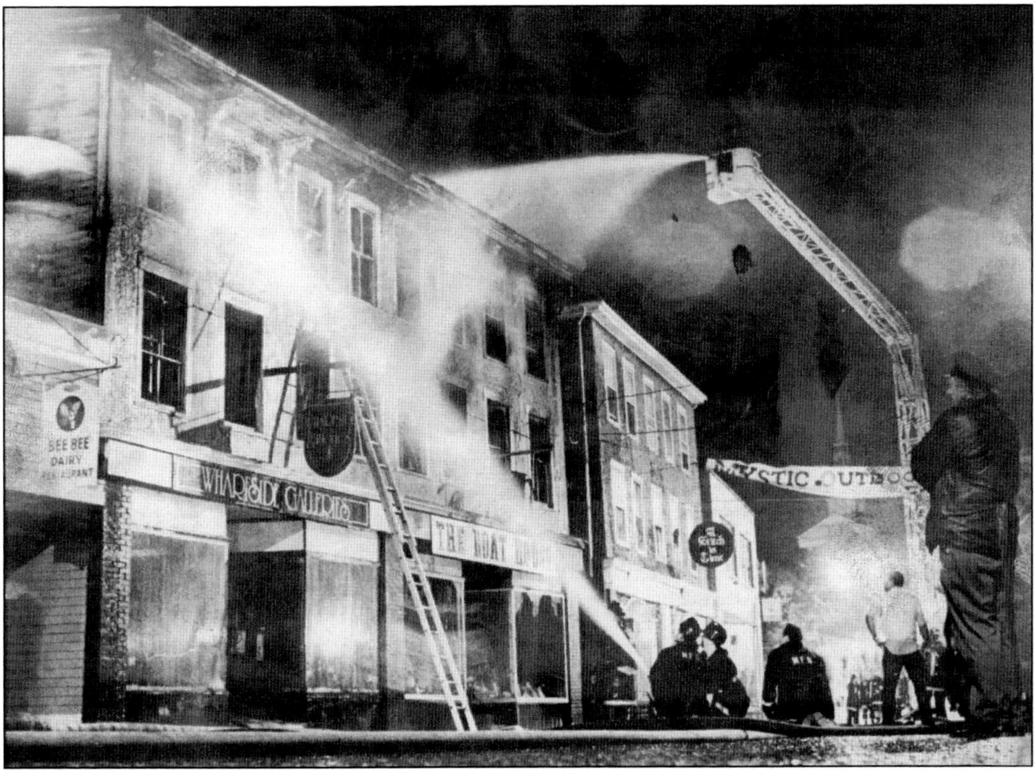

A New London man pleaded guilty to second- and third-degree arson for causing this fire at 39–41 West Main Street on August 6, 1974. After breaking into the building and failing to find money to steal, the man decided to torch the building, heavily damaging it and affecting the adjoining structures. (Mystic Fire Department.)

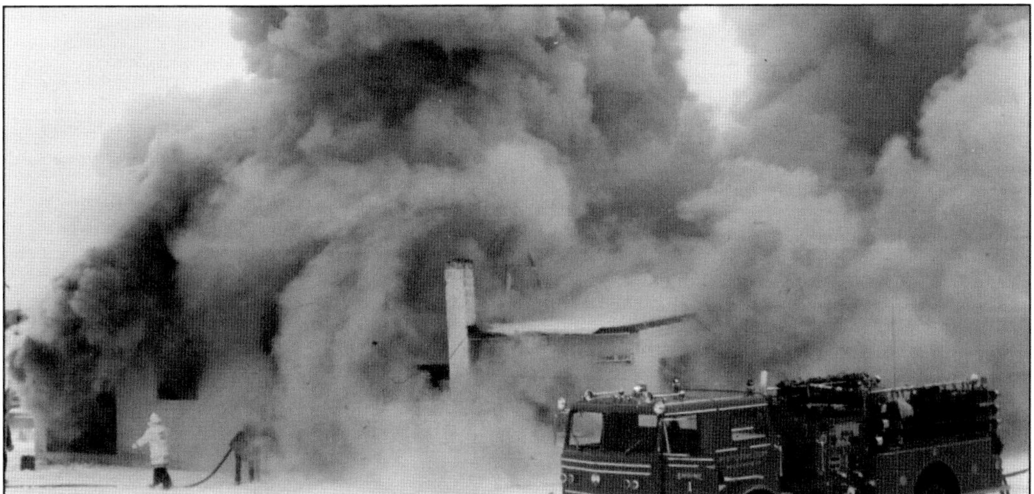

On February 24, 1972, fire chief Albert Brooks and assistant chief Tom Tetlow led Mystic's fire crews as they worked to fight a fire at the Mystic Shipyard at Willow Point. The fire was extinguished at the opposite end of a building where another fire had caused $100,000 in damage four months earlier. (Mystic Fire Department.)

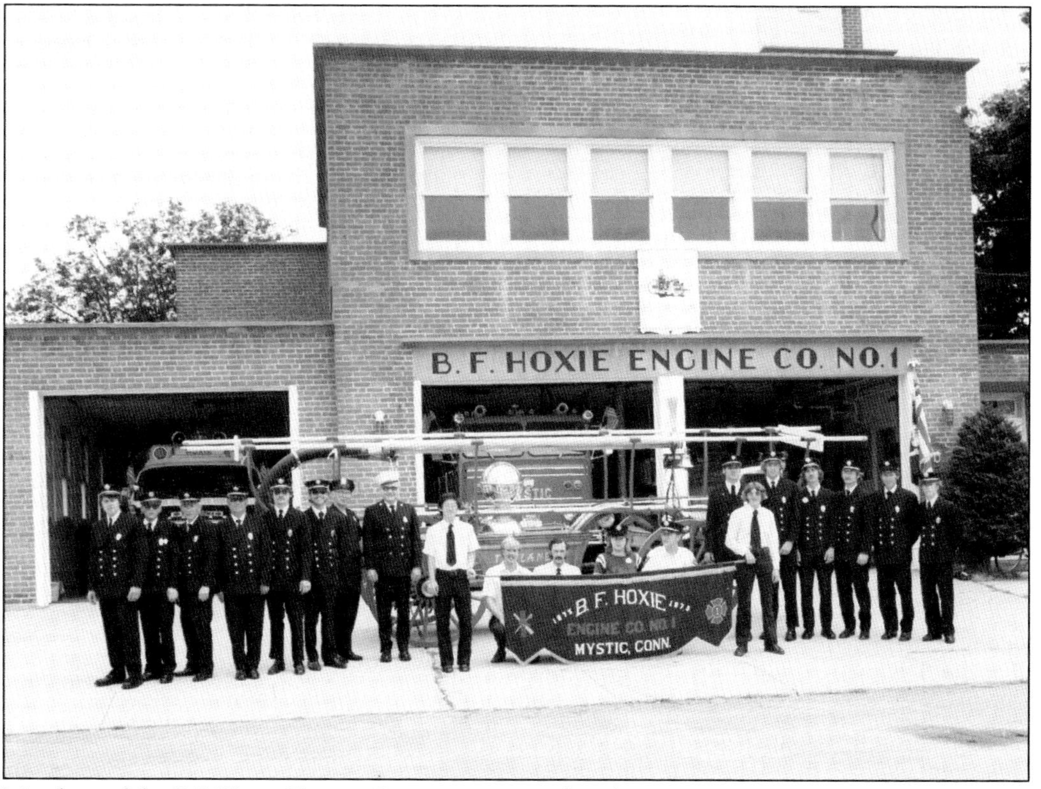

Members of the B.F. Hoxie Engine Company pictured in this c. 1976 image are, from left to right, Davis Smith, Frank Brewer Sr., Charles Main, Robert Marikle, Carl Johnsen, Craig May, Joseph Herman, Frank L. Hilbert, Stanley Ono, David Magin, Richard Nye, Cris Brewer, Edwin Wolff, William Cannon, Randy Noyes, Frank C. Hilbert, Richard Brooks, William Peterson, Robert Peters, and Frank Brewer. (Mystic Fire Department.)

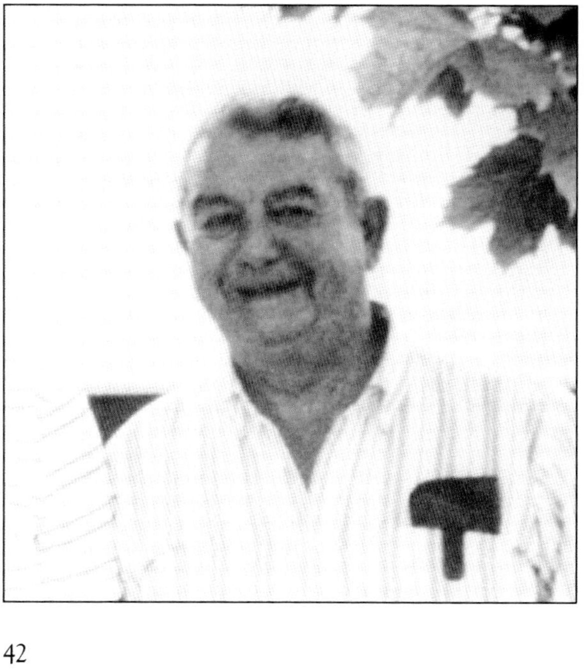

On December 5, 1989, firefighter Russell Musante Sr. collapsed from a heart attack while fighting a brush fire behind the Mystic Ice Building on New London Road. Musante was rushed to Lawrence + Memorial Hospital, where he passed away. Musante was 69 years old and a 44-year veteran of the Mystic Hook and Ladder Company. (Russell Musante Jr.)

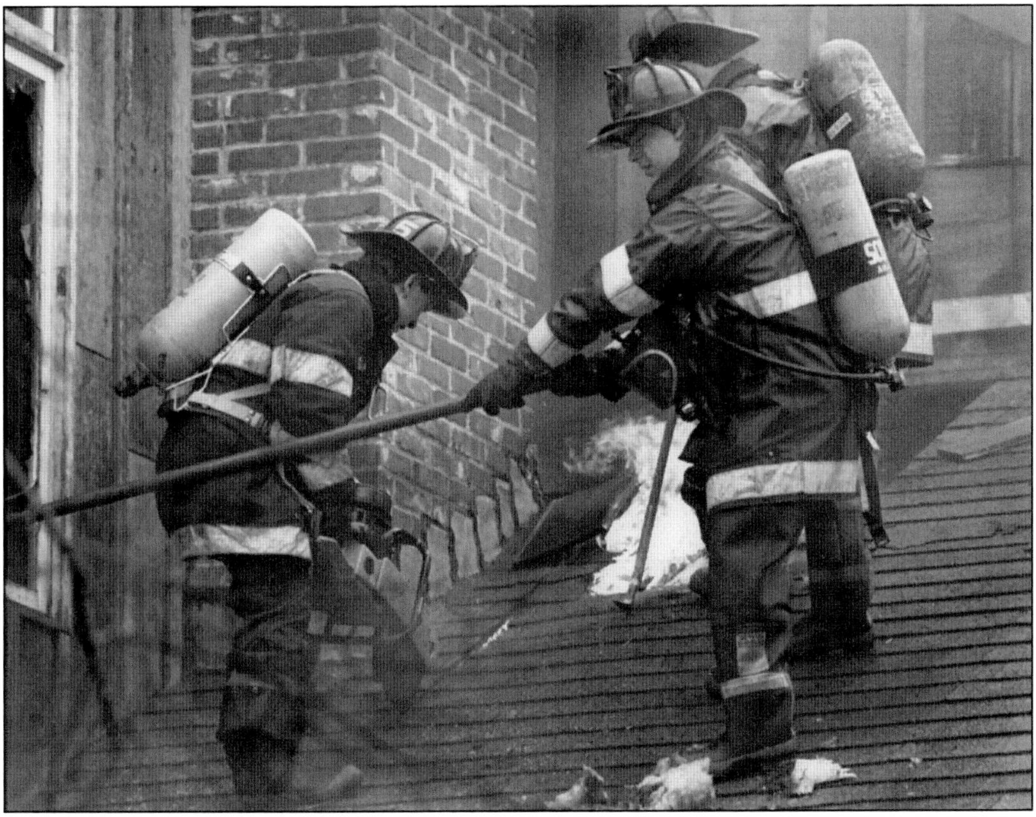

In this c. 1988 photograph, members of the Mystic Hook and Ladder Company perform ventilation operations at a structure fire. From left to right are Mike Lindy, Scott Lindy, and Russell Musante Jr. (behind Lindy). (Mystic Fire Department.)

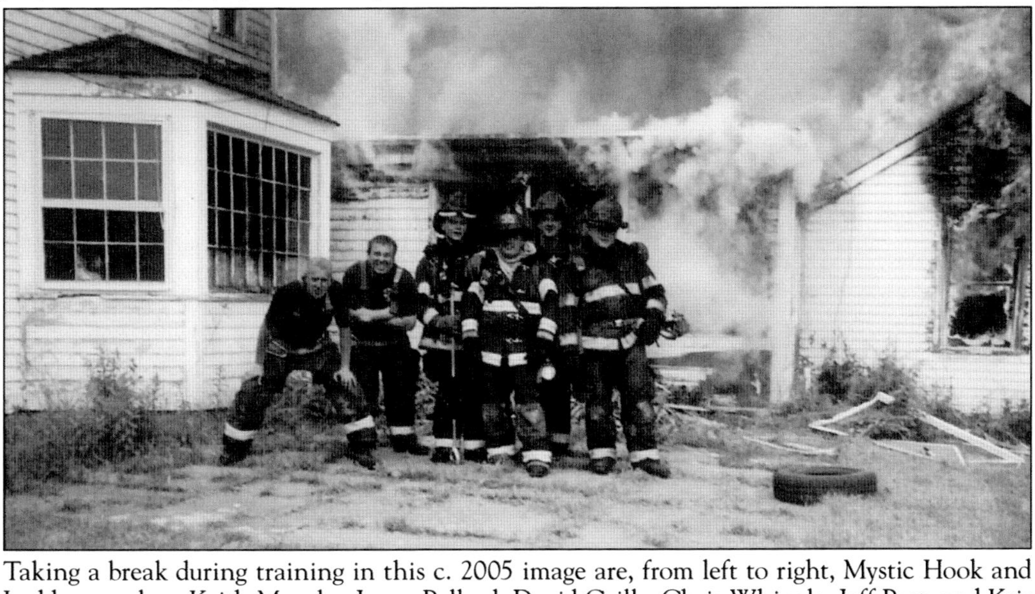

Taking a break during training in this c. 2005 image are, from left to right, Mystic Hook and Ladder members Keith Murphy, Jason Pollard, David Grills, Chris Whipple, Jeff Post, and Kris Grills. (Mystic Fire Department.)

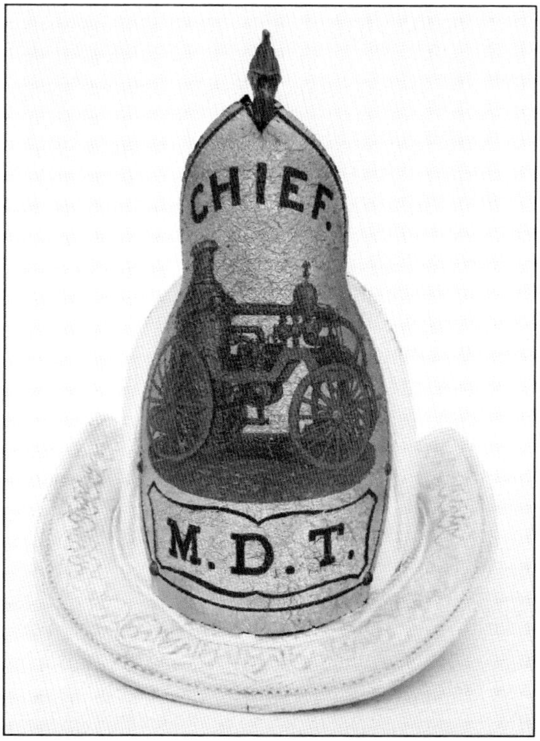

In 1869, Lt. Minthorn D. Tompkins was first recipient of the James Gordon Bennett Award, the Fire Department of New York's highest medal of valor. He retired because of an injury and moved to Mystic with his family. There, Tompkins became a member of the B.F. Hoxie Engine Company, later leaving to help form the Mystic Hook and Ladder Company. He is believed to have served as chief of the department; pictured here is the "high eagle" fire helmet worn by Tompkins when he served as chief. (William Tischer.)

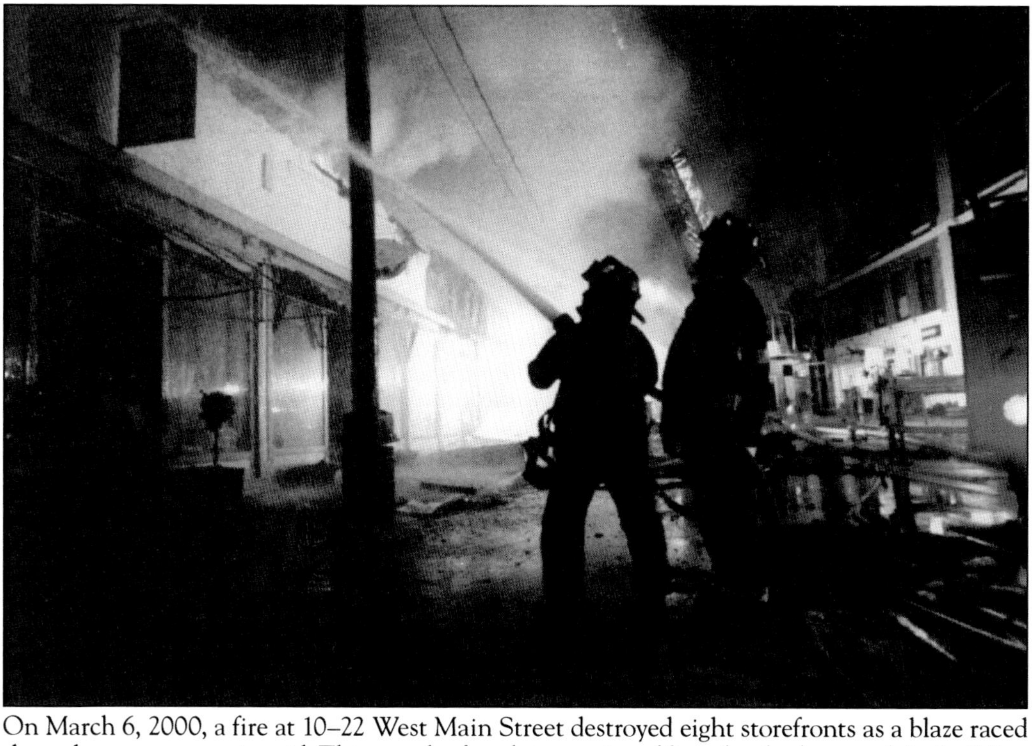

On March 6, 2000, a fire at 10–22 West Main Street destroyed eight storefronts as a blaze raced through a common attic void. This was the fourth in a series of fires that had ravaged the building since 1863. (Mystic Fire Department.)

Prior to the 1930s, fires in the village of Poquonnock Bridge were fought using the bucket brigade system. In June 1934, residents petitioned to establish a volunteer fire company. A few months later, the Poquonnock Bridge Volunteer Fire Department Company No. 1 was organized. Later that year, they purchased a secondhand REO fire truck, which was stored in a garage near Depot Road. In 1941, the company constructed a fire station on Fort Hill Road and hired its first paid driver. Today, the department is comprised of a full staff of paid firefighters and is housed in newer facilities on Long Hill Road. (Poquonnock Bridge Fire Department.)

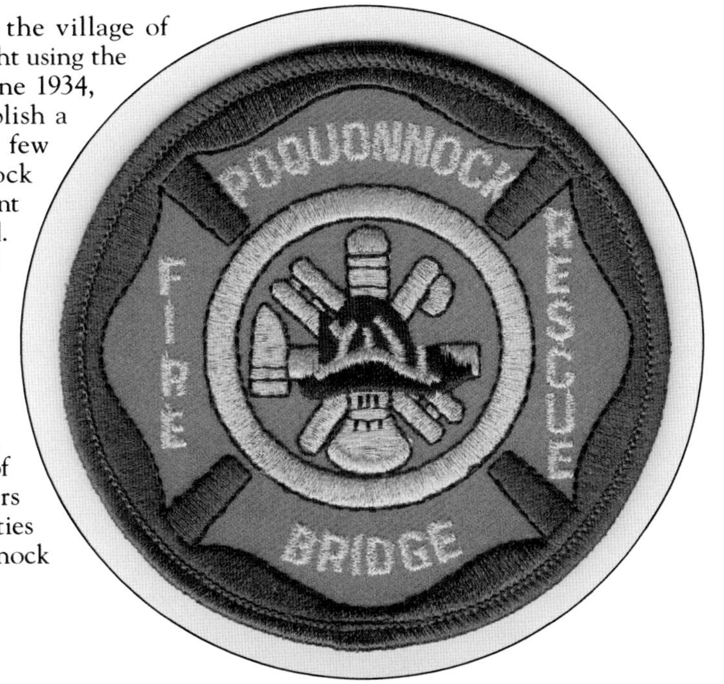

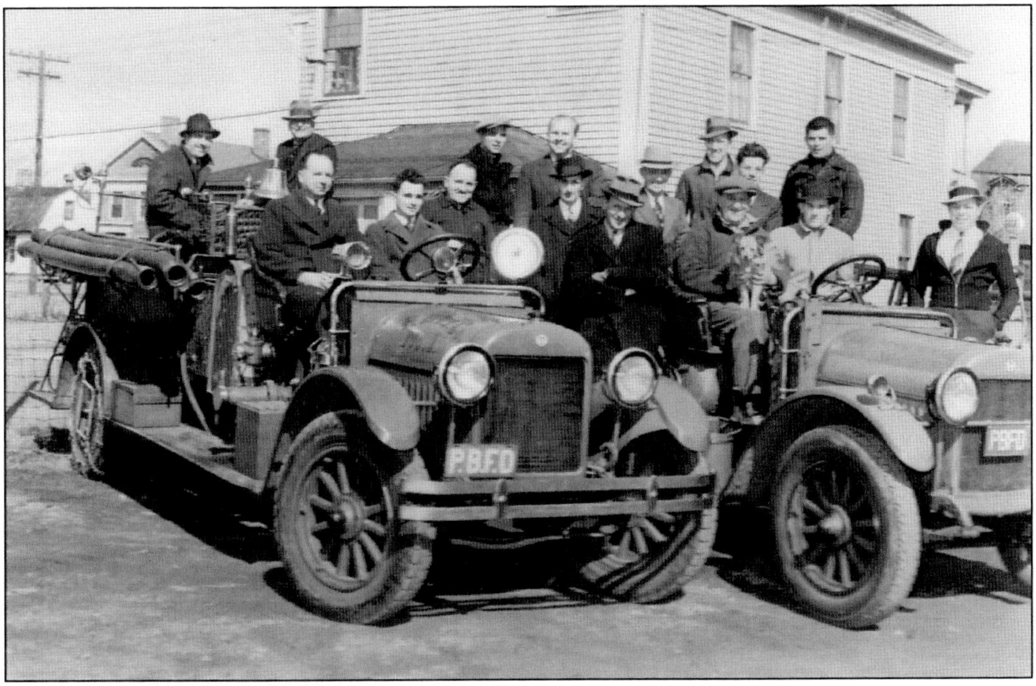

This c. 1940 photograph shows members of the Poquonnock Bridge Volunteer Fire Company posed with the company's two 1925 REO fire trucks. From left to right are Robert Y. Chapman, Joel M. Kenyon, Lewis M. Cromwell, Stuart E. Rowland, Revere E. Clapp, Clair C. Lester, Stanley R. Trail, Edward Weeks, Clarence L. Forbes, Mack F. Schwatlow, Alpheus I. Nye, Joey H. Kenyon, James D. Weeks, Frank J. Pollard, Raymond W. Garlock, and Alger E. Wood. (William Peck, CT Firemen's Historical Society Collection.)

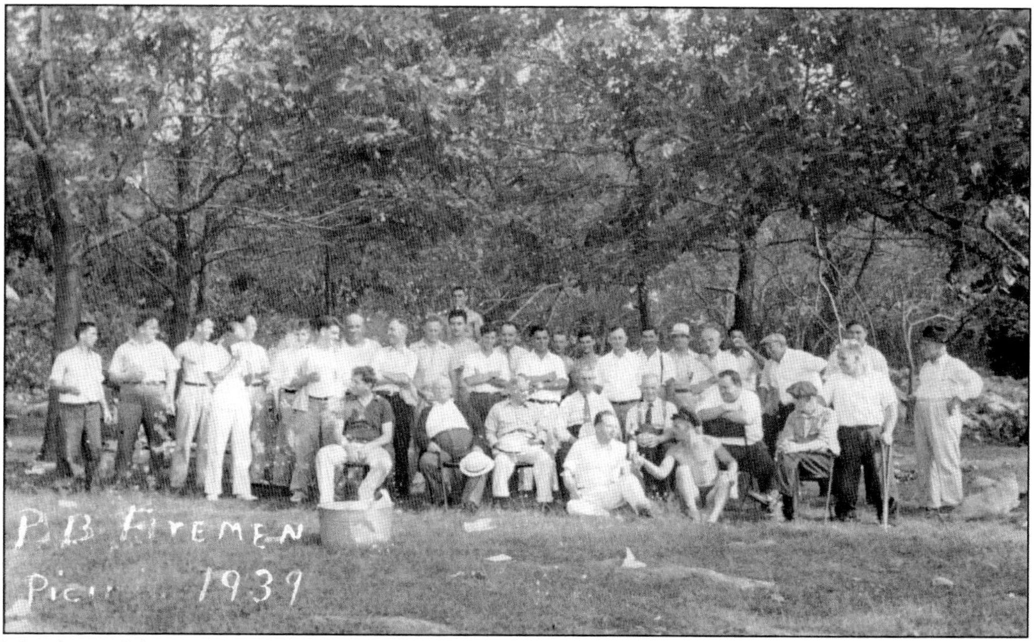

Members of the Poquonnock Bridge Volunteer Fire Company pose during their first-annual picnic in 1939. From left to right are (first row) Robert Chapman, George Vassar, unidentified, William Trail, Lewis Cromwell (on ground), Frank Pollard, unidentified, Leander Lewis, and Charles Tubbs; (second row) unidentified, Sam Johnson, Clifford Marquardt, Clair Lester, Charles Sawyer, John Irving, Cecil Burrows, Stanley Trail, and Charles Edwards; (third row) unidentified, James Edwards, two unidentified, Robert Kilpatrick, Robert Turner, Elbert Chapman, Robert Lewis, Martin Holloway, Revere Clapp, Carl Sawyer, and William Kilpatrick. (Joe Baril.)

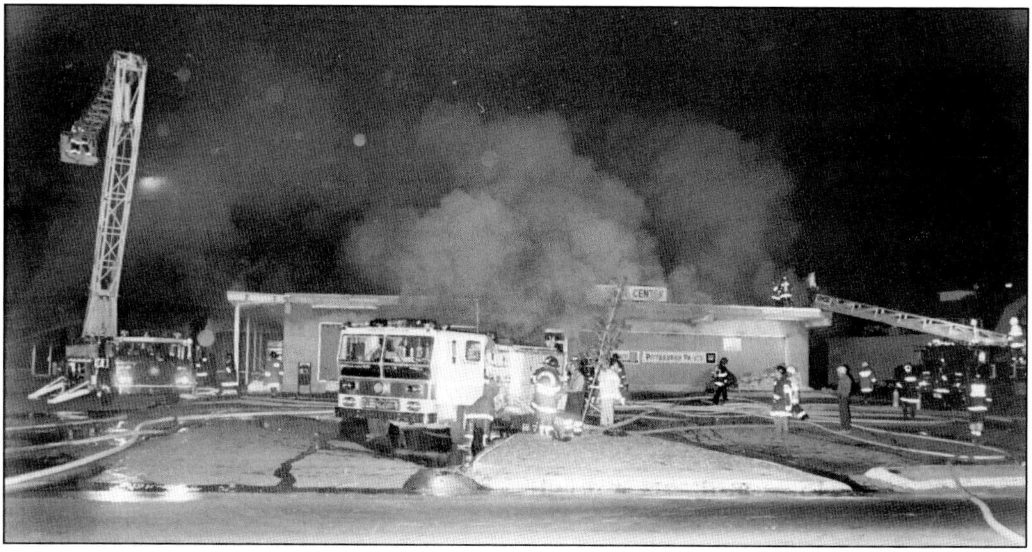

On May 27, 1981, at approximately 11:30 p.m., the Poquonnock Bridge Fire Department responded to a fire at the Johnson's Hardware and Home Center. Within a short period of time, all of Groton's fire departments, as well as departments from surrounding communities, had been requested to assist. The building was totally destroyed, and firefighters were still hosing down smoldering debris at noon the following day. (Joe Baril.)

Firefighter Russell H. Jones Jr., a 20-year veteran of the Poquonnock Bridge Fire Department, suffered a heart attack after returning from a fire alarm on March 16, 1985, and subsequently died on April 1, 1985. Jones had served as a patrolman with the Town of Groton Police Department for 10 years before becoming employed with the Poquonnock Bridge Fire Department. (Joe Baril.)

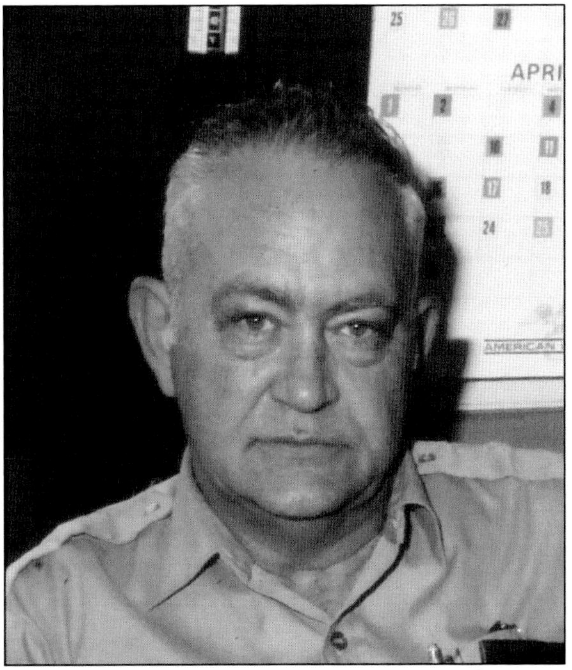

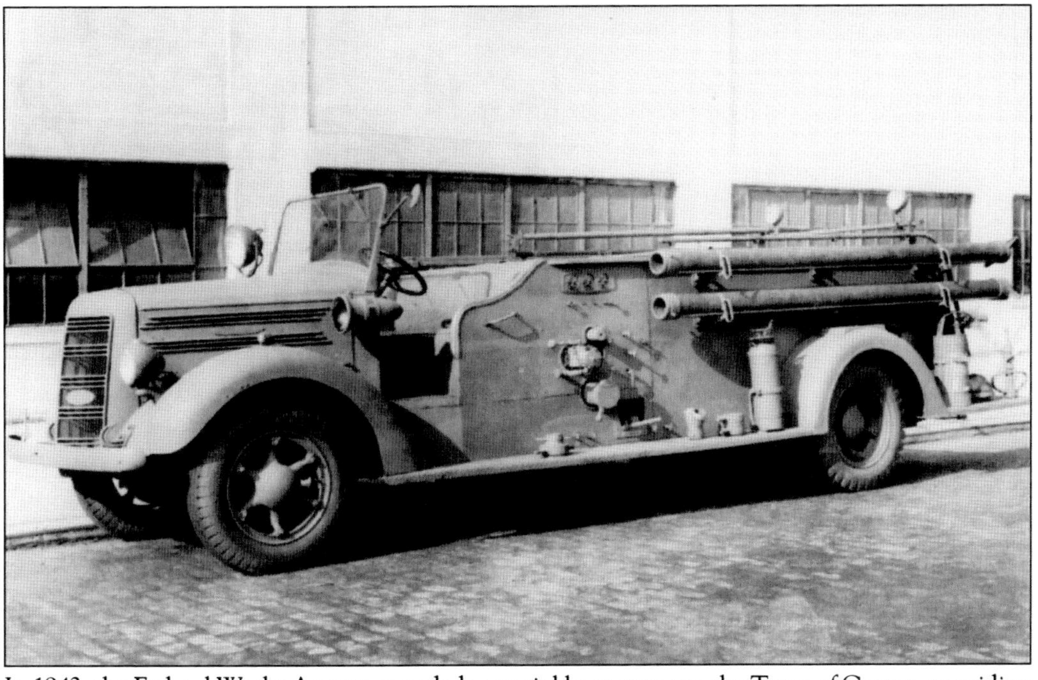

In 1943, the Federal Works Agency awarded a special lease grant to the Town of Groton, providing them with a used 1942 Mack 500-gallon-per-minute pumper fire truck and 1,000 feet of hose to ensure fire protection to the newly constructed, federally funded Fort Hill Homes housing project in Poquonnock Bridge. In 1946, the vehicle was purchased by the Poquonnock Bridge Fire Department, which then was responsible for fire protection of Fort Hill Homes. Pictured here around 1948 is a 1942 Mack truck, painted its original olive green, of the same model as the Town of Groton would have received it in 1943. (Rob Palmer, Connecticut Firemen's Historical Society.)

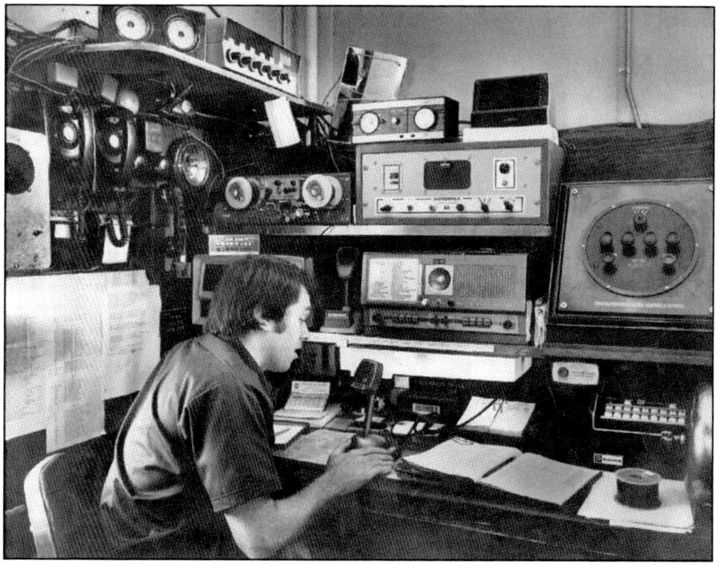

Prior to the Town of Groton establishing the Groton Fire Alarm Dispatch Center in the Town of Groton Police Headquarters, most fire departments in Groton operated their own dispatch centers. This photograph from the late 1970s shows Lt. John Shaw manning the dispatch center, also known as the "Watch Desk," in the Poquonnock Bridge Volunteer Fire Company No. 1 firehouse on Fort Hill Road. (Joe Baril.)

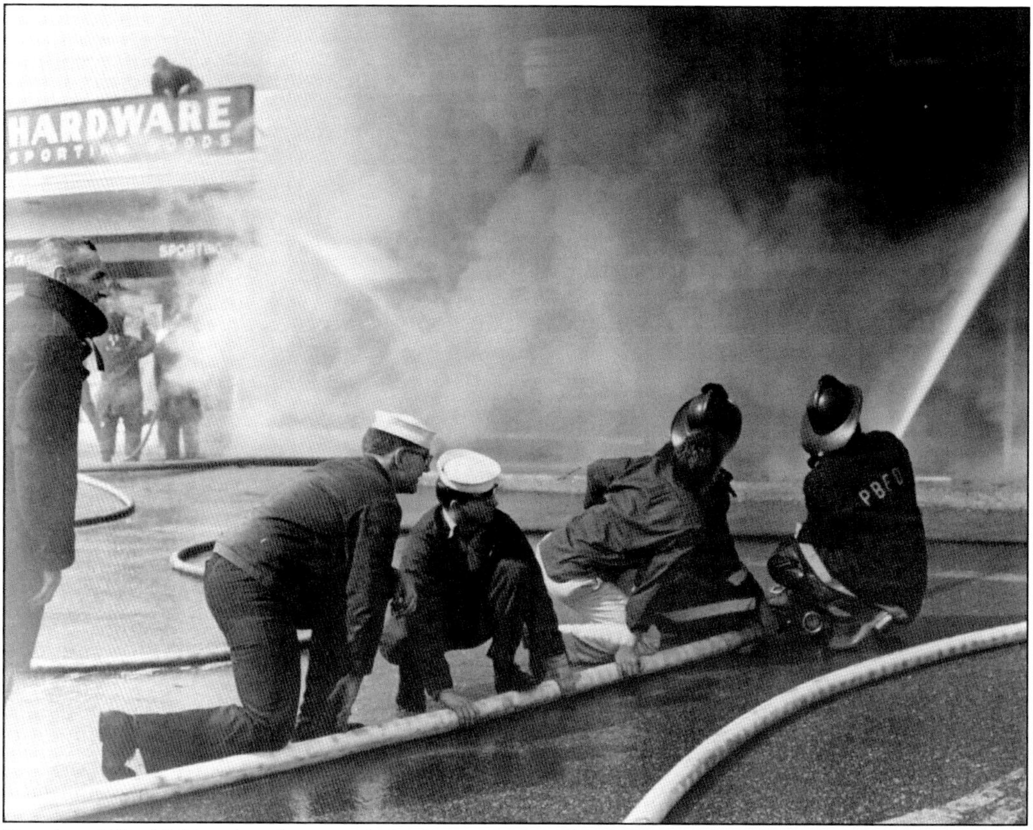

On April 29, 1963, a fire destroyed the First National Food Store located on the south end of a 22-store shopping center on Long Hill Road in Groton. All area fire departments were dispatched to fight the fire, which was brought under control in about an hour. This photograph shows unidentified firemen from the Poquonnock Bridge Fire Department and unidentified Navy sailors directing water into the burning building. (Joe Baril.)

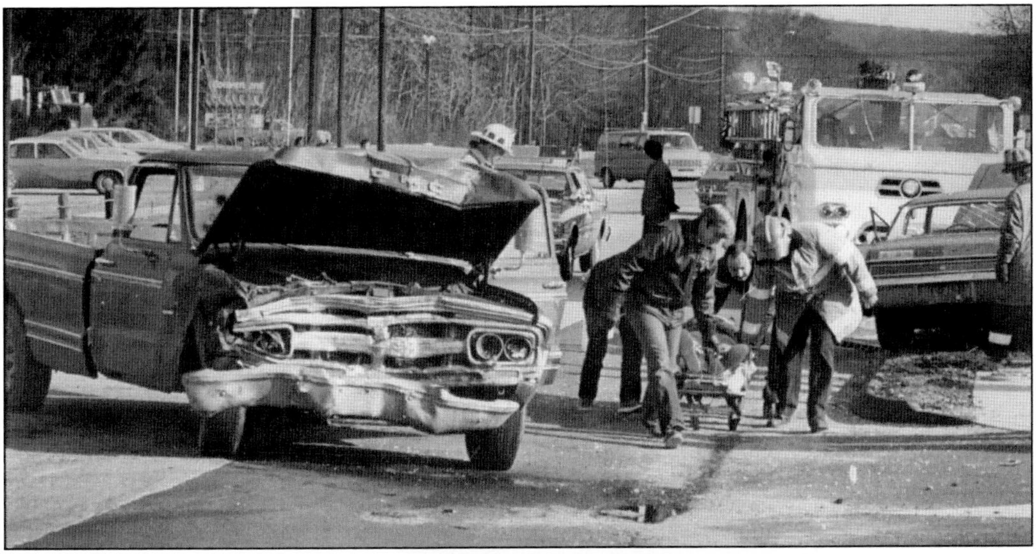

Poquonnock Bridge Fire Department firefighters and other emergency service personnel attend to injured persons at a two-vehicle accident that occurred in front of the Auto Emissions Center on Route 184 in Groton on January 4, 1983. (Joe Baril.)

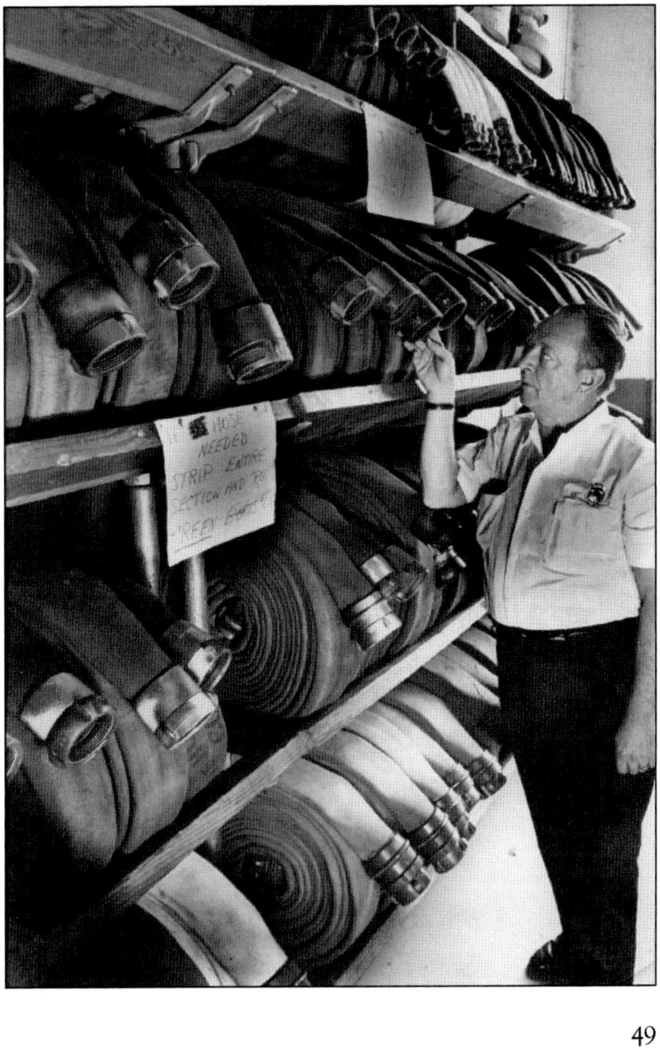

Carl Sawyer, former chief of the Poquonnock Bridge Fire Department, conducts a routine inspection of fire hoses at the Fort Hill station in this c. 1975 picture. Sawyer, who retired in 1978 after serving as chief for 24 years, had been a member of the department since its inception in late 1930s. (Joe Baril.)

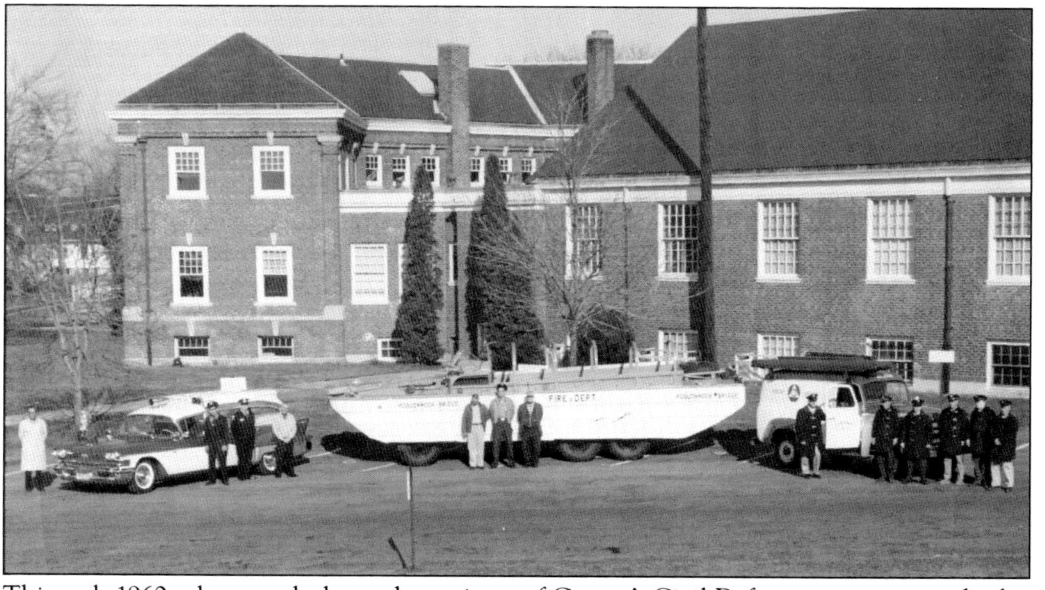

This early-1960s photograph shows three pieces of Groton's Civil Defense apparatus on display at the Groton Town Hall. From left to right are members of the Groton Ambulance Association with their newly acquired ambulance, firefighters from the Poquonnock Bridge Fire Department in front of their land-and-sea duck, and firefighters from the City of Groton in front of their rescue truck. (Joe Baril.)

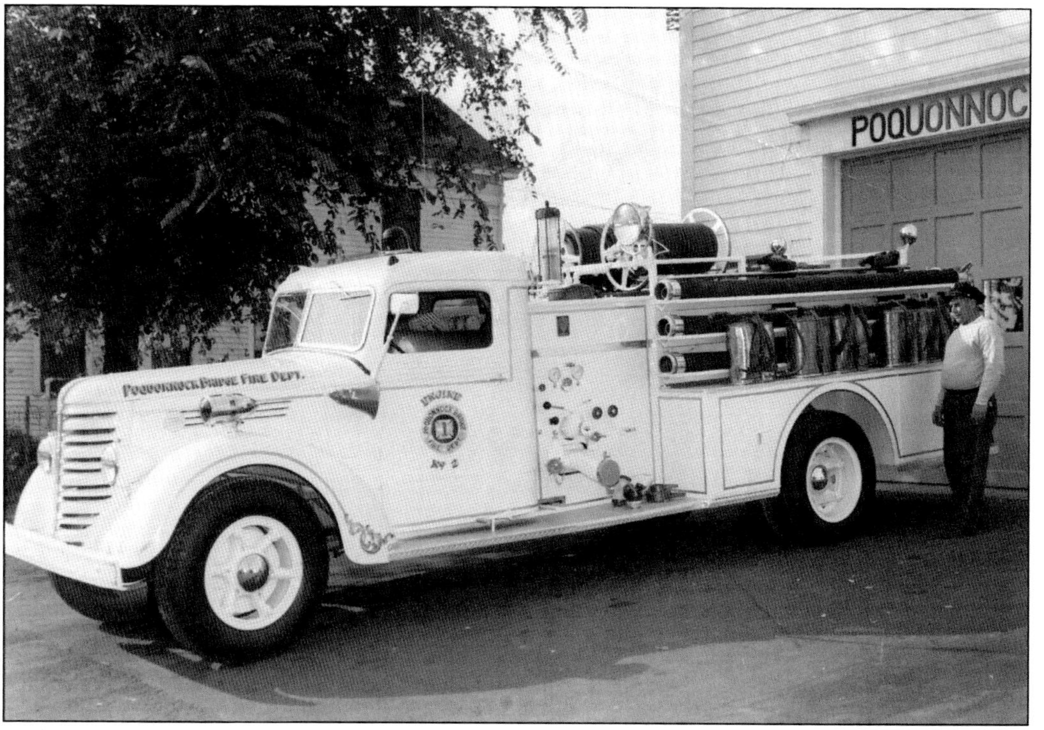

In this July 1955 photograph, an unidentified volunteer with the Poquonnock Bridge Fire Department is standing next to the company's Engine No. 2, a 1948 Federal pumper truck. The vehicle is parked in front of the Poquonnock Bridge firehouse on Fort Hill Road. (Joe Baril.)

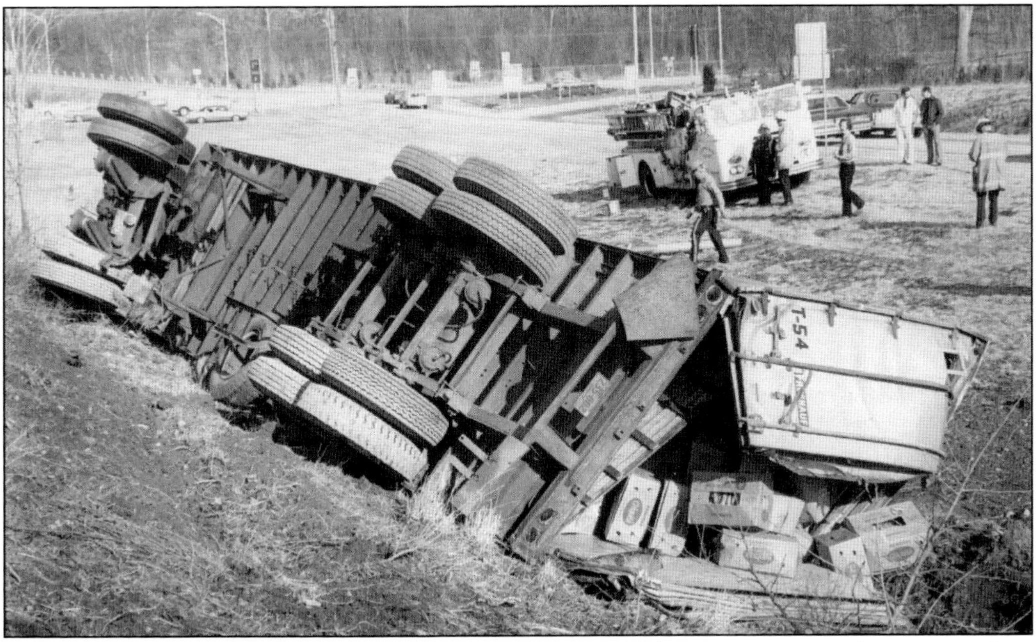

Poquonnock Bridge firefighters and Connecticut State Police troopers are shown providing emergency assistance at a tractor-trailer accident that occurred near Exit 88 of Interstate 95 in Groton on April 15, 1980. (Joe Baril.)

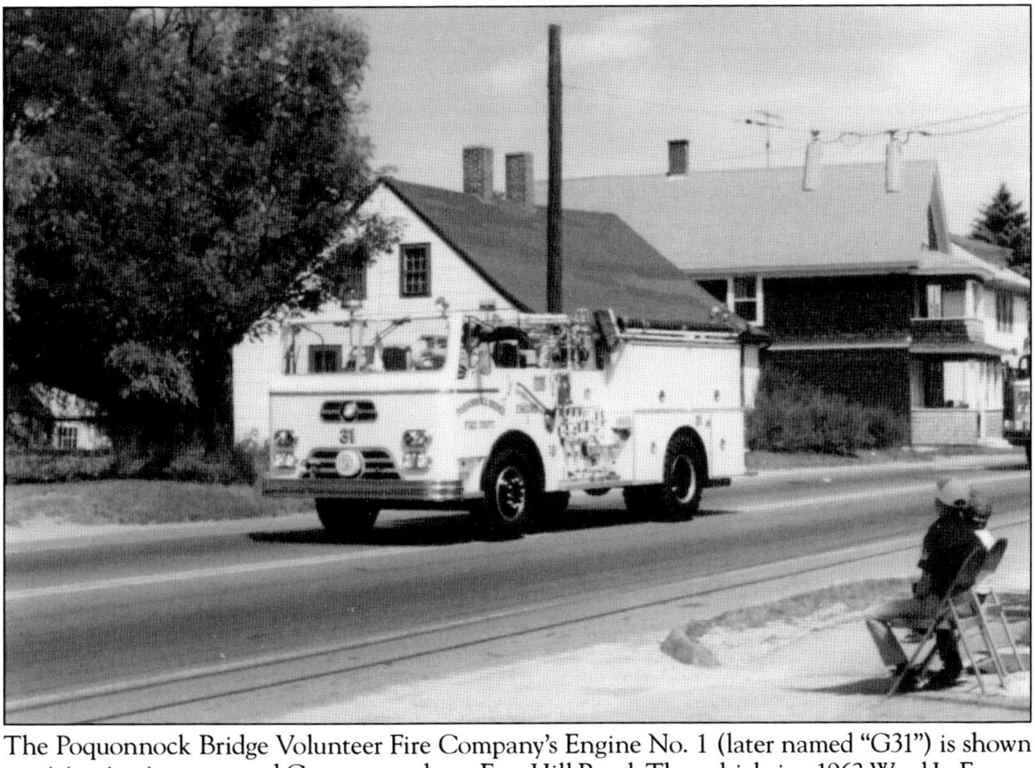

The Poquonnock Bridge Volunteer Fire Company's Engine No. 1 (later named "G31") is shown participating in an annual Groton parade on Fort Hill Road. The vehicle is a 1962 Ward LaFrance 1,000-gallon-per-minute pumper truck. (Joe Baril.)

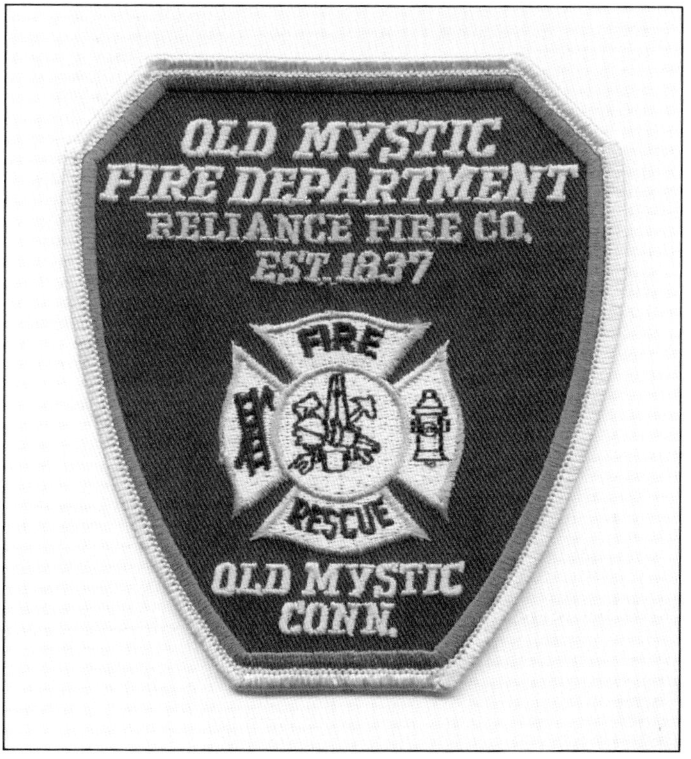

A concerned citizen named John Hyde spearheaded the organization of the New Reliance Hose Company in 1837 after a large fire in Stonington. After some lean years, it was reorganized as the Reliance Fire Company in 1942. After state legislation was passed in 1962, the Old Mystic Fire District was born, and the Old Mystic Fire Department continues to serve the area today. (Old Mystic Fire Department.)

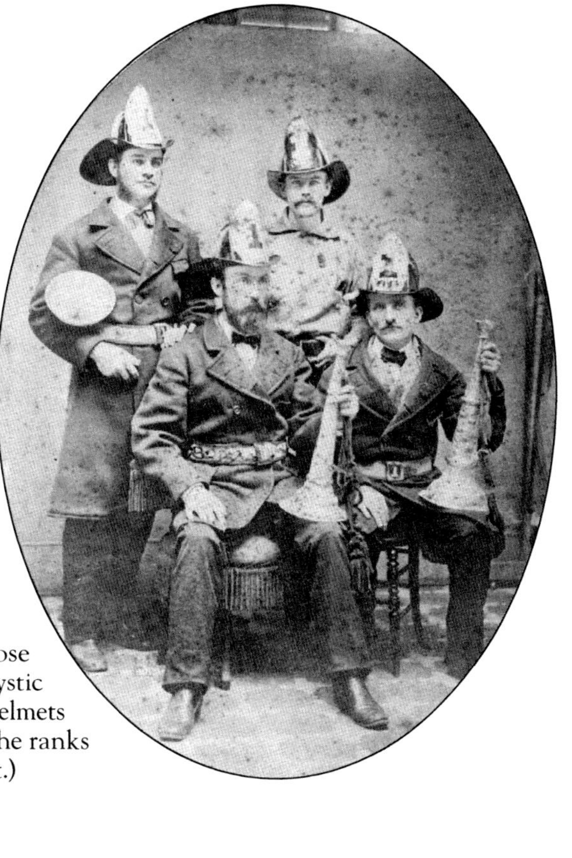

The founding officers of the Reliance Hose Company sit for a photograph. The Old Mystic Fire Department still possesses several of the helmets and belts shown here; these items denoted the ranks of the officers. (Old Mystic Fire Department.)

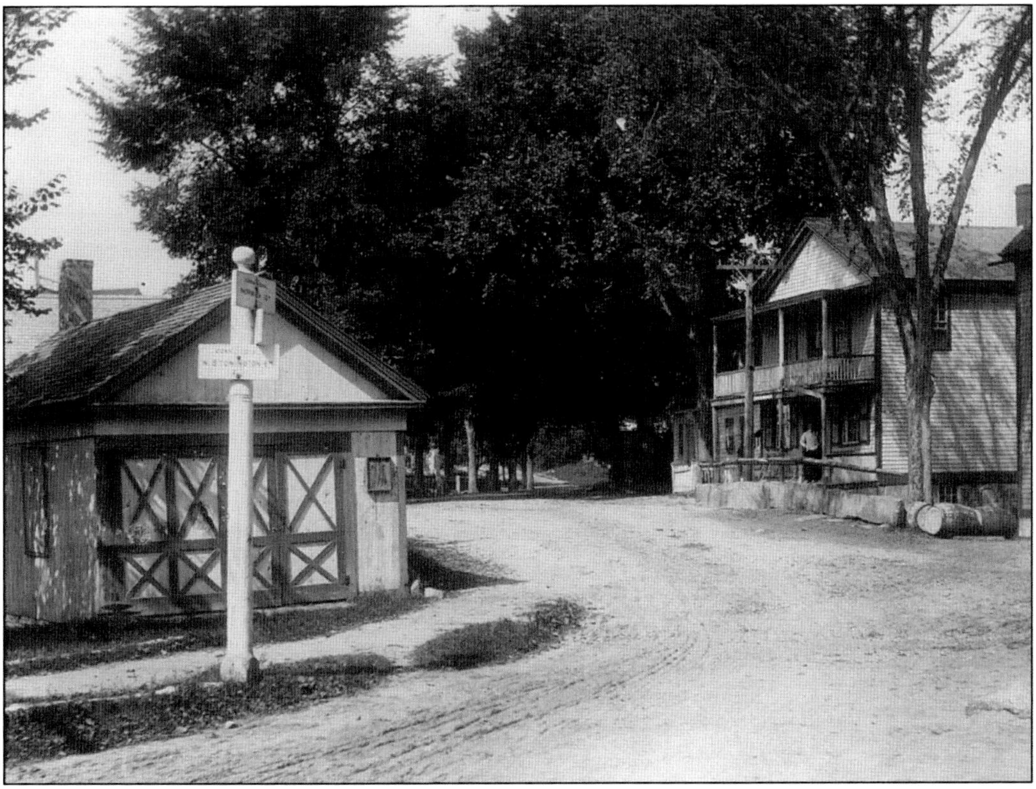

The garage on the left in this c. 1925 photograph was the home of the original Reliance Hose Company at the intersection of Route 27 and Main Street. The fire station is now gone, as is the building to the right, which burned down in the early 1960s. (Old Mystic Fire Department.)

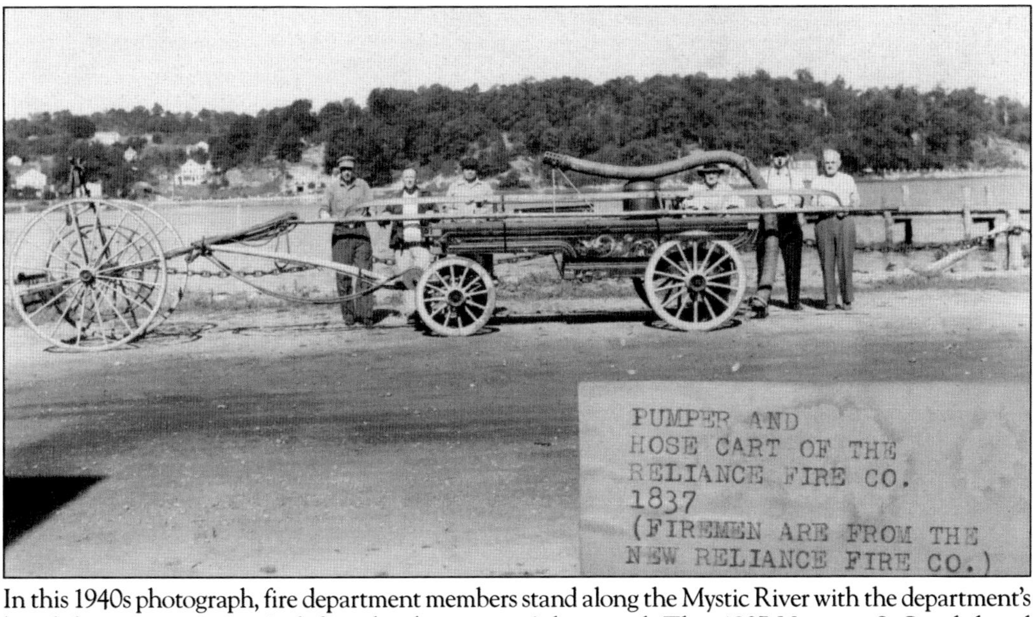
PUMPER AND
HOSE CART OF THE
RELIANCE FIRE CO.
1837
(FIREMEN ARE FROM THE
NEW RELIANCE FIRE CO.)

In this 1940s photograph, fire department members stand along the Mystic River with the department's hand-drawn apparatus. At left is the department's hose reel. This 1837 Vanness & Smith hand pumper (also known as a hand tub) was made in New York. (Old Mystic Fire Department.)

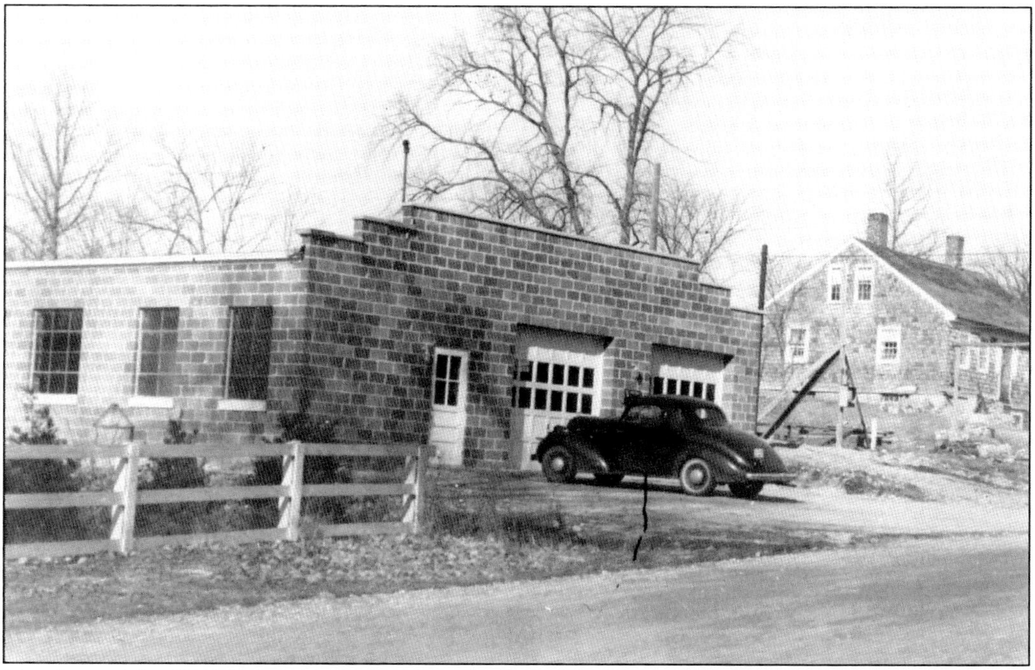

Members of the Old Mystic Fire Department built this cinder block station at 21 North Stonington Road in 1941; this picture was taken soon after it was completed. Later, a second floor was added to the building, which remained in use until 1999, when it was torn down. A new station was erected on the same site and is still in use today. (Old Mystic Fire Department.)

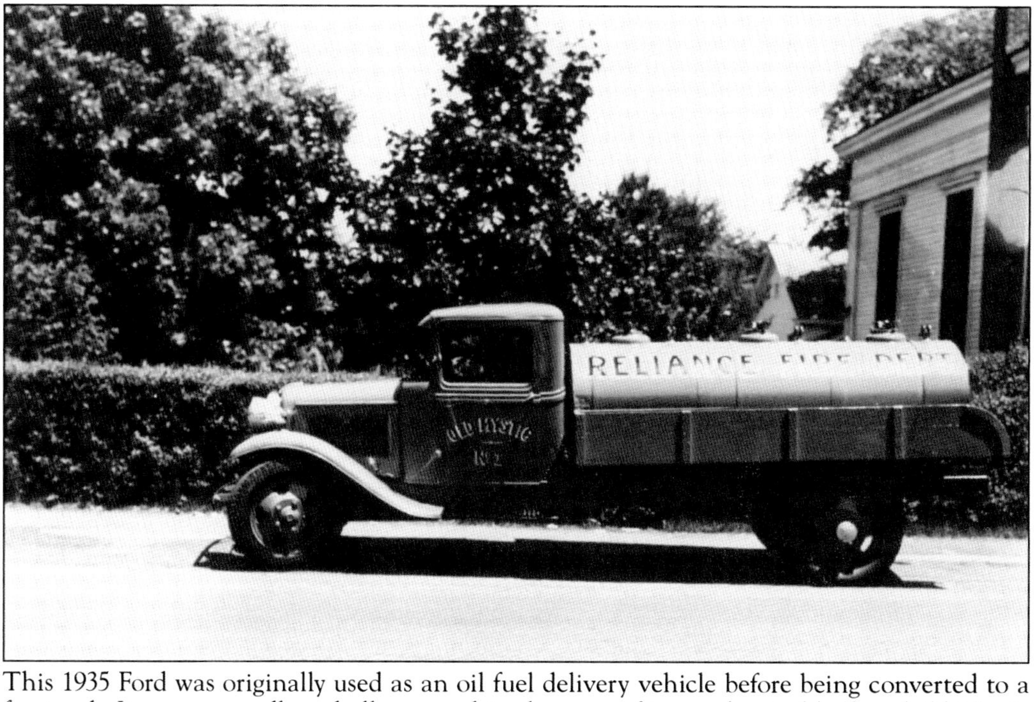

This 1935 Ford was originally used as an oil fuel delivery vehicle before being converted to a fire truck. It was reportedly a challenge to drive because of its mechanical brakes. (Old Mystic Fire Department.)

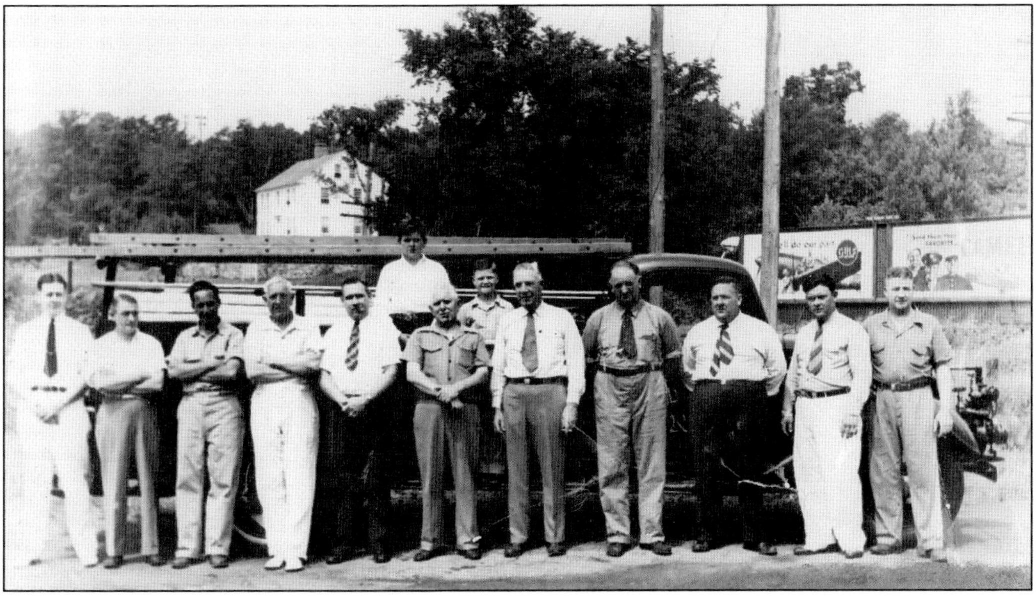

Charter members of the Reliance Fire Company pose with their 1937 Chevrolet engine in the early 1940s. After years of sparse activity, a reorganization in 1942 stimulated growth in the company that became the foundation of today's department. (Old Mystic Fire Department.)

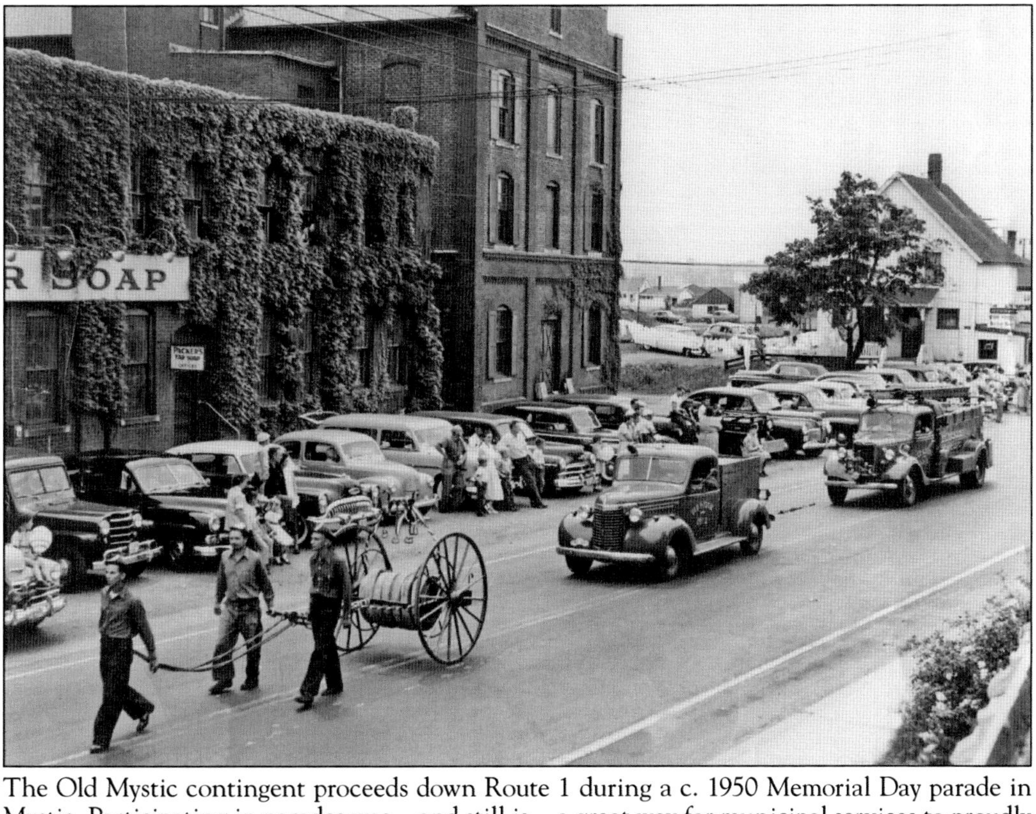

The Old Mystic contingent proceeds down Route 1 during a c. 1950 Memorial Day parade in Mystic. Participating in parades was—and still is—a great way for municipal services to proudly display their apparatus to the public. (Joe Baril.)

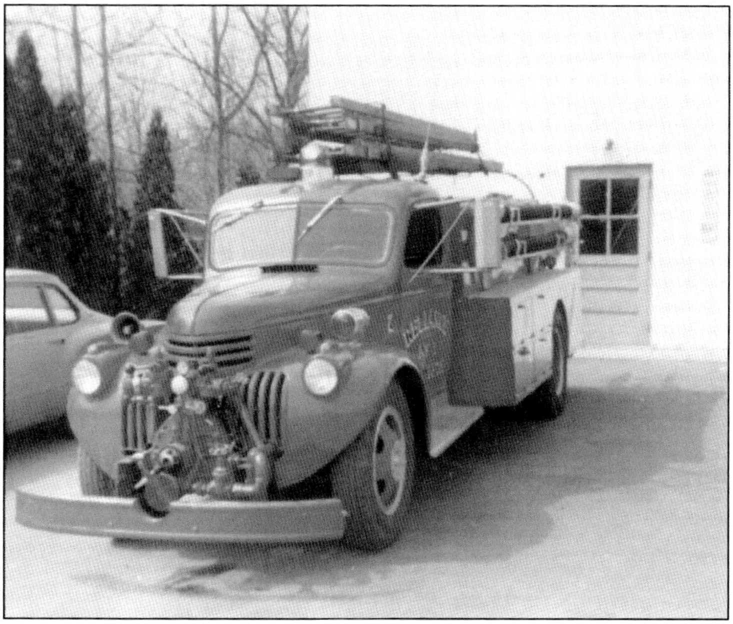

This 1937 Chevrolet is parked in front of Station No. 1. The vehicle, modified by department members, had a 500-gallon-per-minute pump, and its ladders were stored on an overhead rack above the hose bed. (Old Mystic Fire Department.)

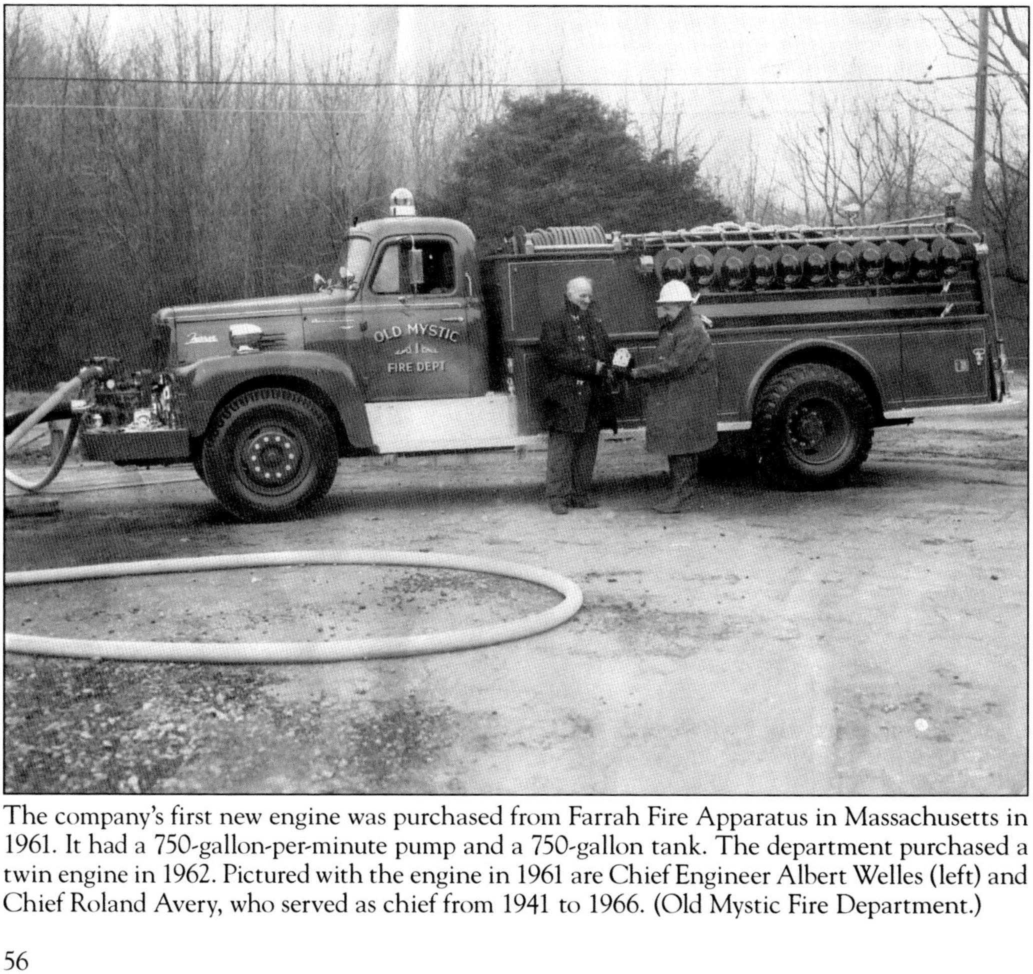

The company's first new engine was purchased from Farrah Fire Apparatus in Massachusetts in 1961. It had a 750-gallon-per-minute pump and a 750-gallon tank. The department purchased a twin engine in 1962. Pictured with the engine in 1961 are Chief Engineer Albert Welles (left) and Chief Roland Avery, who served as chief from 1941 to 1966. (Old Mystic Fire Department.)

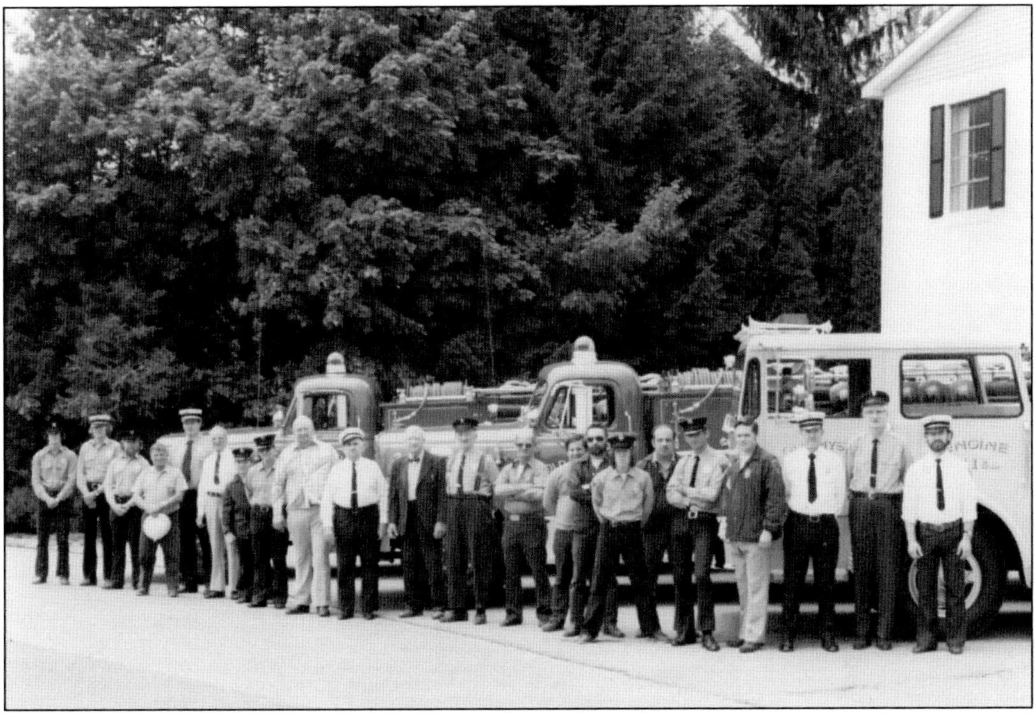

Company members pose for a group photograph in 1976. From left to right are Fred Dewick, Carl Hewitt, Tom Fox, Russ Williams, William Welles Jr., Aldo Lena, Ken Brimlow, Richard Brimlow, Red Wooster, Roland Avery, Horace Williams, Albert Welles, Charles Emery, Dan Hall, Tim Sullivan, Wade Chapman, Ed Ryan, Bruce Reid, Charles Larkin, Chief Ed Hanks, William Welles Sr., and Richard Green. (Old Mystic Fire Department.)

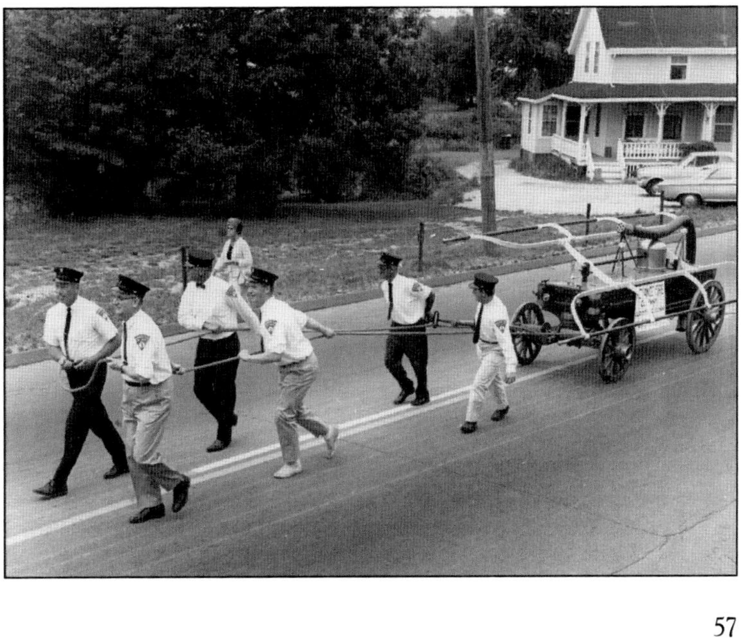

Company members pull their hand pumper through a Memorial Day parade in Mystic in the 1960s. The early hand pumpers were smaller and could be carried by four men. Some were mounted on skids and dragged to the fire. An apparatus with wheels made mobility considerably easier. (Old Mystic Fire Department.)

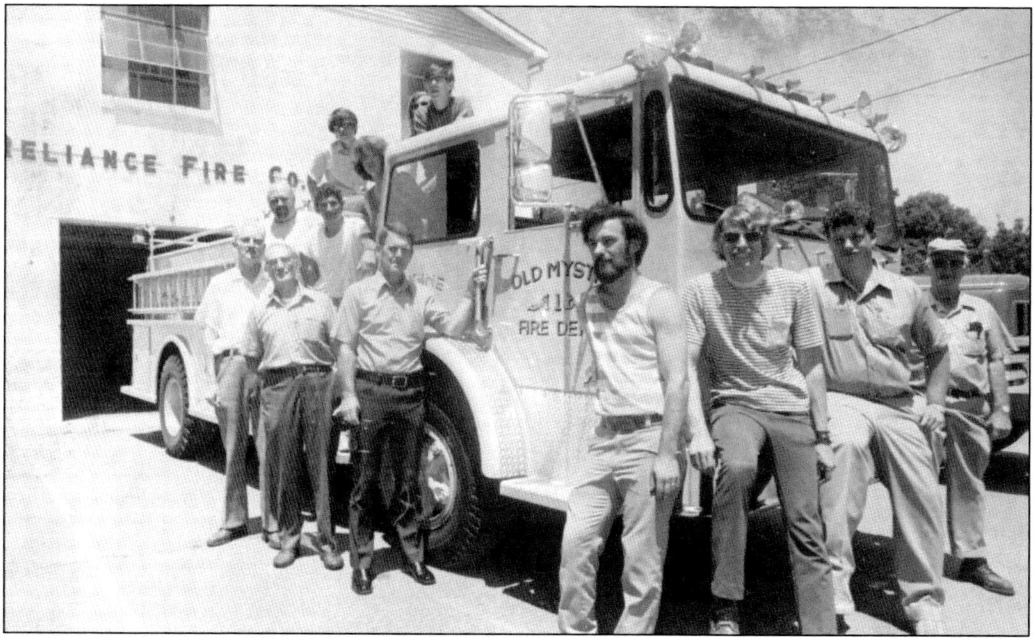

Members pose with the district's 1975 Farrah 1,000-gallon-per-minute engine. From left to right are (standing) William Welles Sr., Aldo Lena, Chief Ed Hanks, Richard Green, Carl Hewitt, William Welles Jr., and ? Austin; (on steps) Red Wooster, Bruce Reid, and Ken Richards Jr.; (on top) Tom Fox, Wade Chapman, and an unidentified member. (Old Mystic Fire Department.)

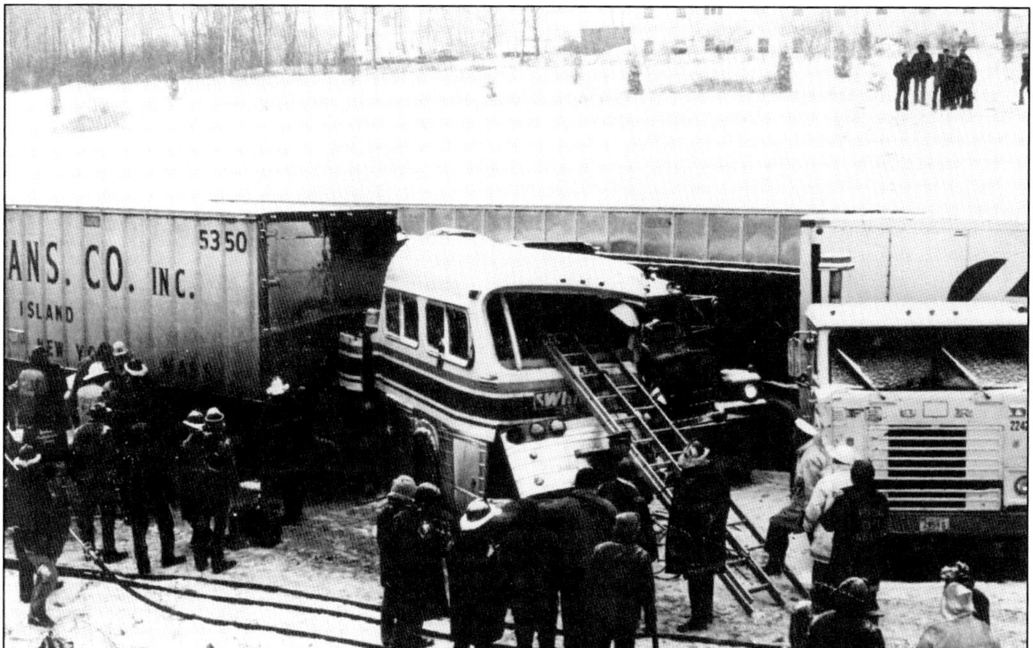

On February 8, 1974, a bus carrying a New Jersey college basketball team was crushed between two tractor-trailers in an accident at exit 89 on Interstate 95 in Old Mystic. The team captain and his wife were trapped inside the bus for about 90 minutes before they were rescued. (Old Mystic Fire Department.)

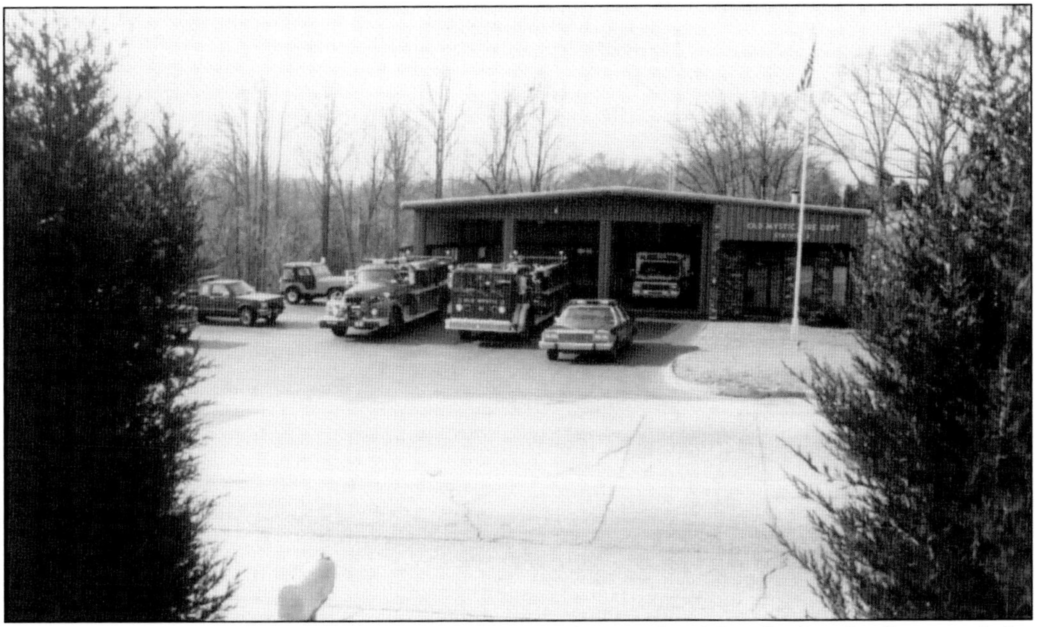

The original Station No. 2, built in 1979, is pictured around 1986 with the chief's car and the 1962 and 1975 Farrah engines parked outside. Pictured inside the Old Mystic Fire Department station is a Mystic River Ambulance Association ambulance that was temporarily housed there while the ambulance association built their own facilities. (Old Mystic Fire Department.)

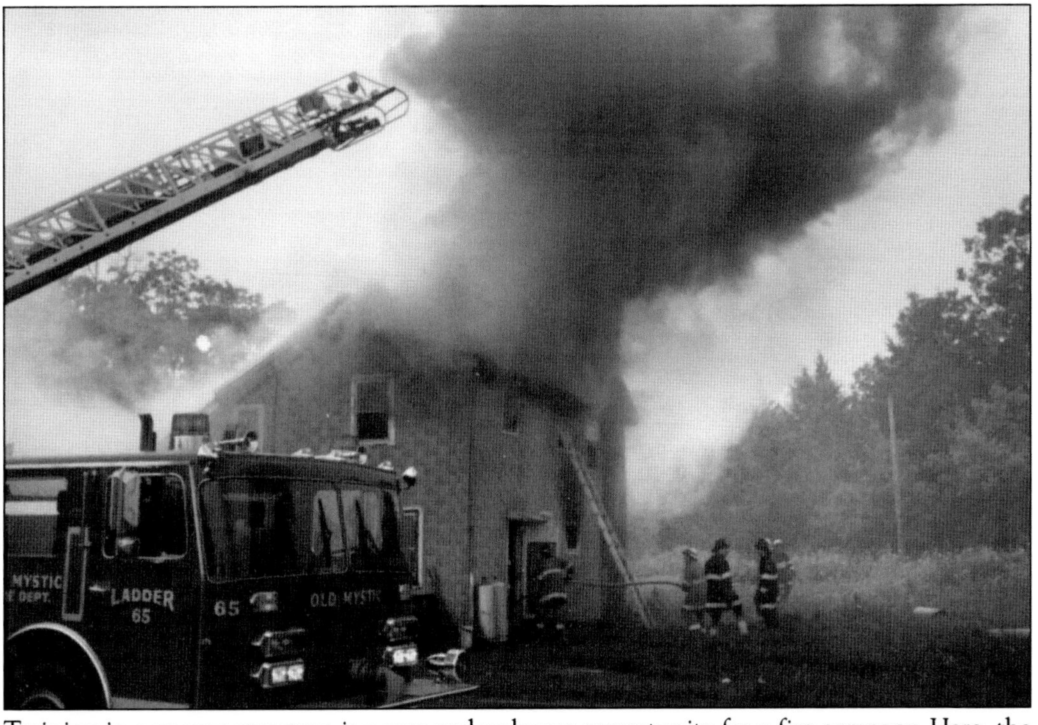

Training in a vacant structure is a rare and welcome opportunity for a fire company. Here, the Old Mystic crews utilize a structure at the corner of Routes 184 and 117, where the Bess Eaton doughnut shop was located. (Old Mystic Fire Department.)

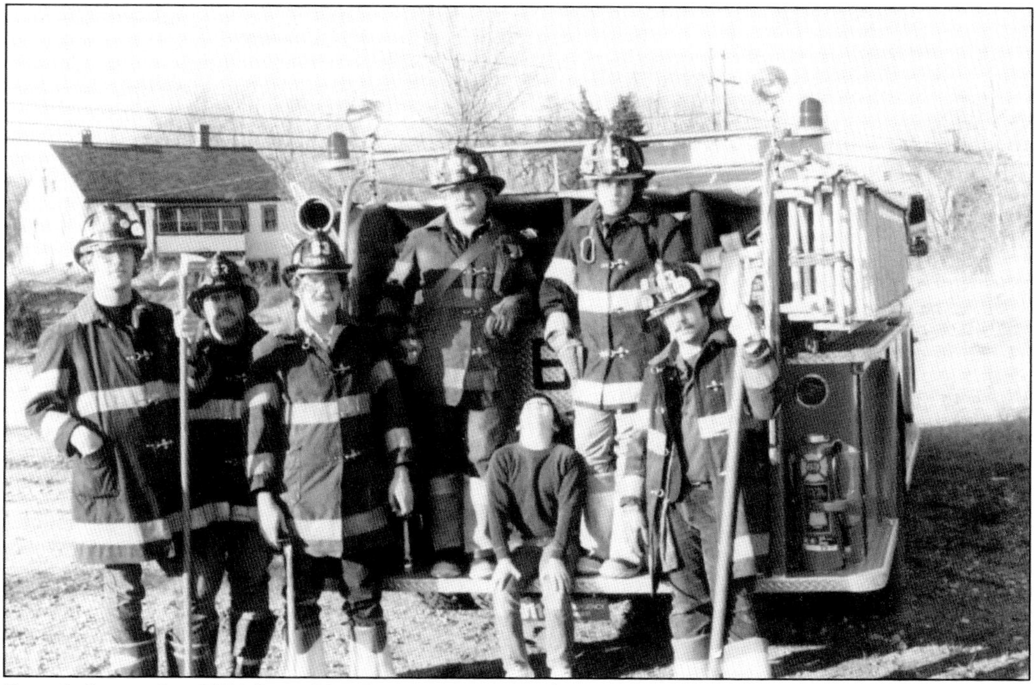

From left to right, Old Mystic Fire Department members Jim Sanquedolce, David Bogue, William Allen, Zacary Hermann, Rick Ellie, and Mark Beebe stand ready for work at the rear of Engine No. 62. Danny Steel, a friend of the firemen, is seated on the end of the truck. (Old Mystic Fire Department.)

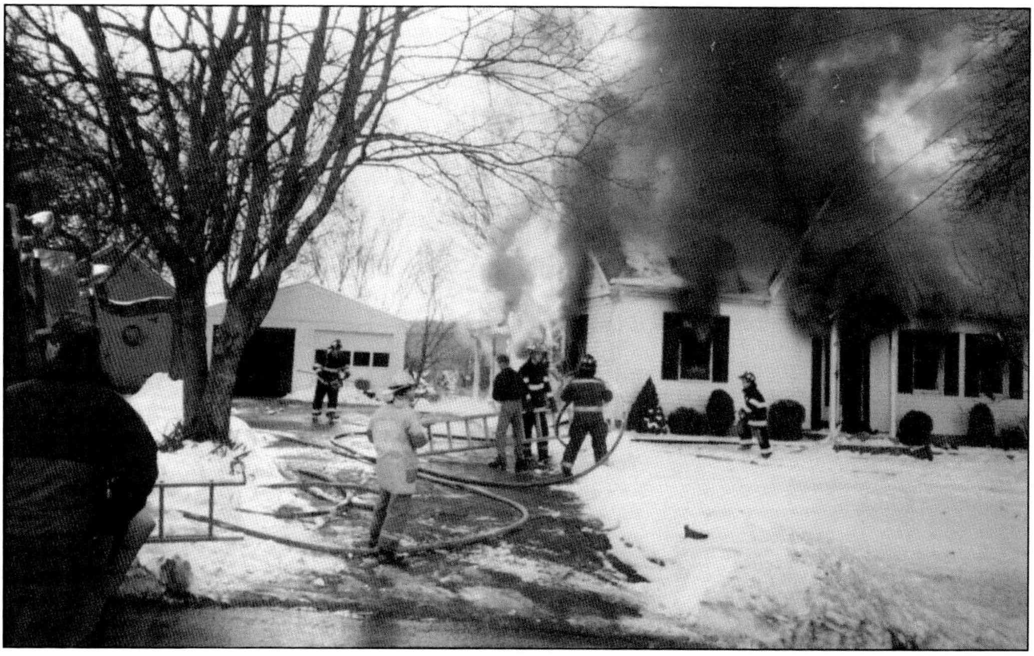

In this c. 1998 photograph, Chief Kenneth Richards Jr. (in light-colored coat) takes command of a structure fire on Whitehall Avenue as the Old Mystic crews prepare to make entry. The fire, which started in the kitchen, was extinguished in short order. (Old Mystic Fire Department.)

The Noank Volunteer Fire Company No. 1 was organized in 1895. At the time, Noank was primarily a fishing village, and boatbuilding was its major industry. Fire was a constant threat due to the use of wood in the construction of boats and buildings in the village, as well as the use of wood and coal for heat. As a major defense for fires, a large water tower was constructed near the center of the village to provide water pressure to the largest boatbuilding yard, the Palmer Shipyard, and to fire hydrants in the center of the village. The first firehouse was located in a large wooden structure on Cedar Street near the Noank Baptist Church's parking lot. The fire company currently occupies more modern facilities on Ward Street. The department is still mostly manned and operated by volunteers. (Noank Fire Department.)

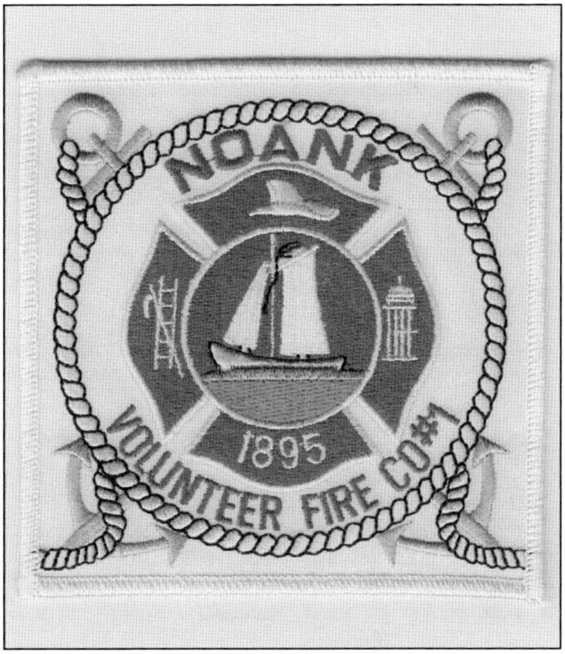

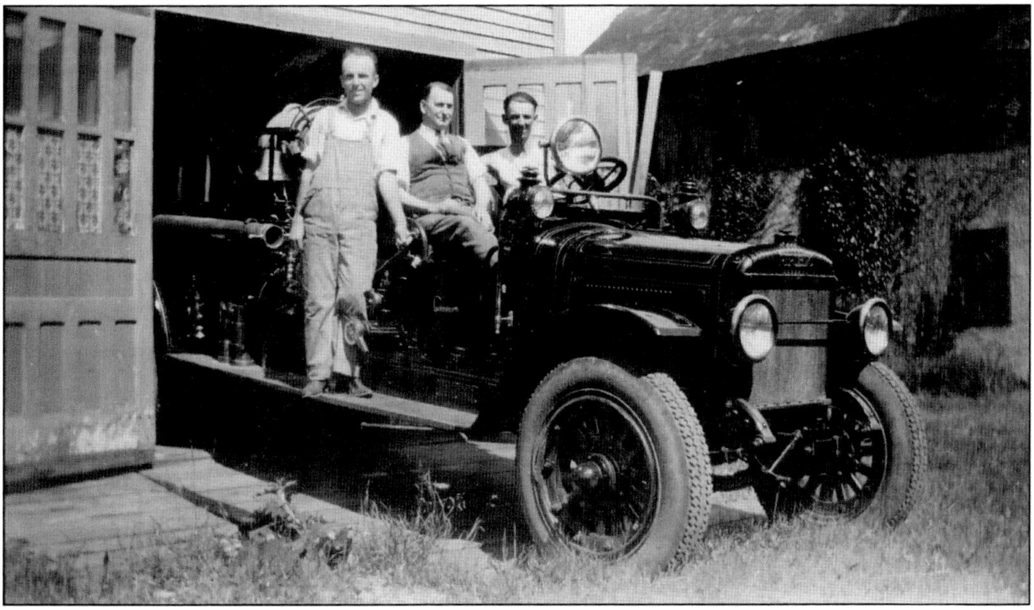

The Noank Fire Department's first motorized firefighting truck, a 1924 Republic pumper, is pictured in front of the old Noank firehouse on Cedar Street. Manning the truck are, from left to right, Hadley Fitch, an unidentified volunteer, and Walter Palmer. (Noank Fire Department.)

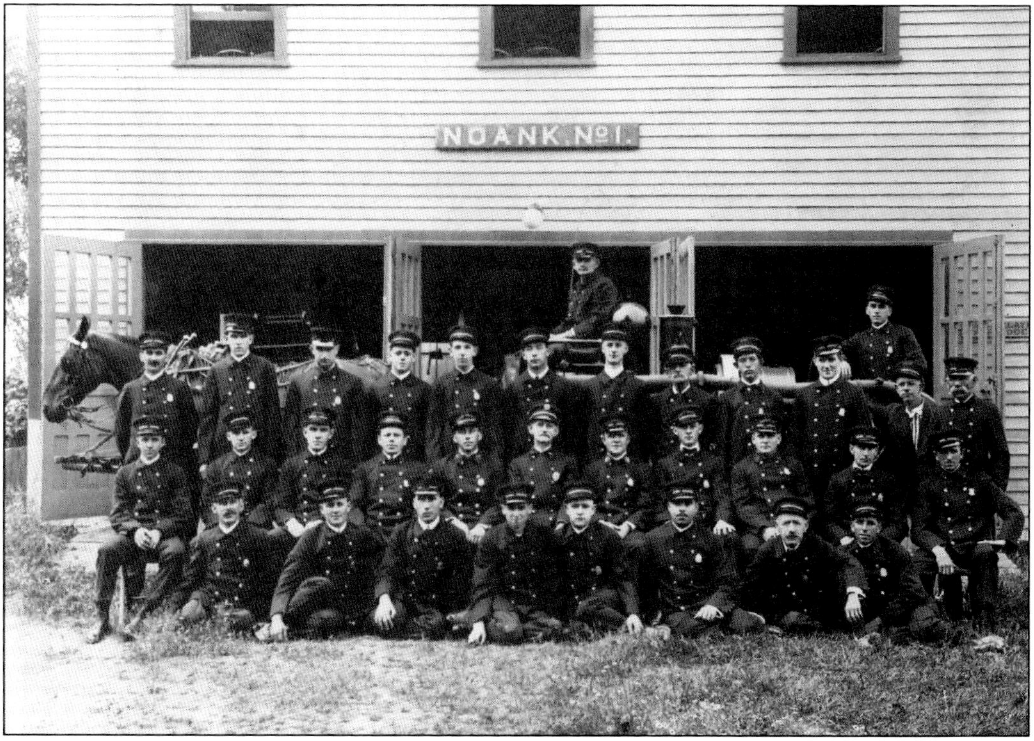

This c. 1920 photograph shows Noank volunteer firefighters posed in front of the old firehouse on Cedar Street. From left to right are (first row) Silas Weaver, Douglass McDonald, Gabe McGaw, Neil Morrison, John McQuarrie, Charles Squadrito, George Brady, and Ira C. Smith; (second row) Eugene Burdick, Fred Fitzpatrick, George W. Brown, John Ellis, James Campbell, Chief L.L. Parks, Charles McDonald, Ivan Crossman, Burt Rathbun, Almond Meister, and Walter Wolverton; (third row) S.B. Patterson, Lloyd C. Brown, Arthur Fitch, Bernard McDonald, Rowland Hill, Alfred Banks, Albert Fitch, Harold Ashbey, Edgar Ashbey, Merton Beebe, Arthur McKenzie, Walter McDonald, Frank Barlow, and Capt. Neal Fowler. The two men in the far background are unidentified. (Noank Fire Department.)

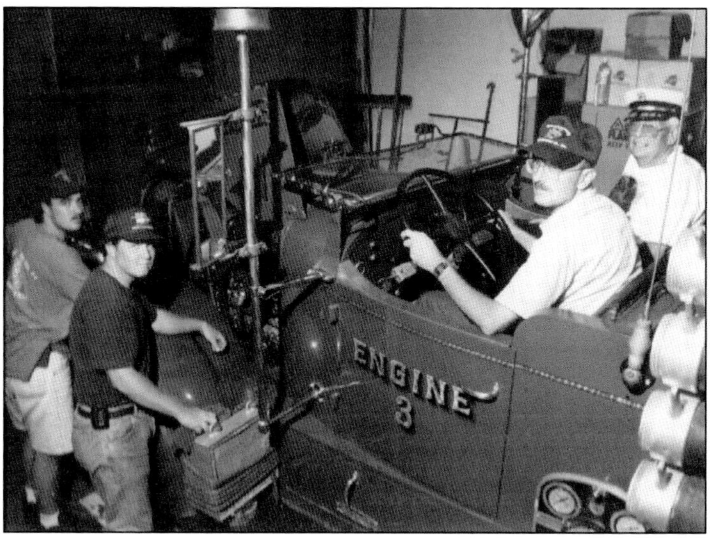

From left to right, Noank volunteer firefighters Mark Ashcraft, Al Beck, Larry Spees, and Dick Latham are pictured inside the current firehouse, located on Ward Street, preparing Engine No. 3, a 1939 Seagrave pumper truck, for the fire department's centennial parade in 1995. (Noank Fire Department.)

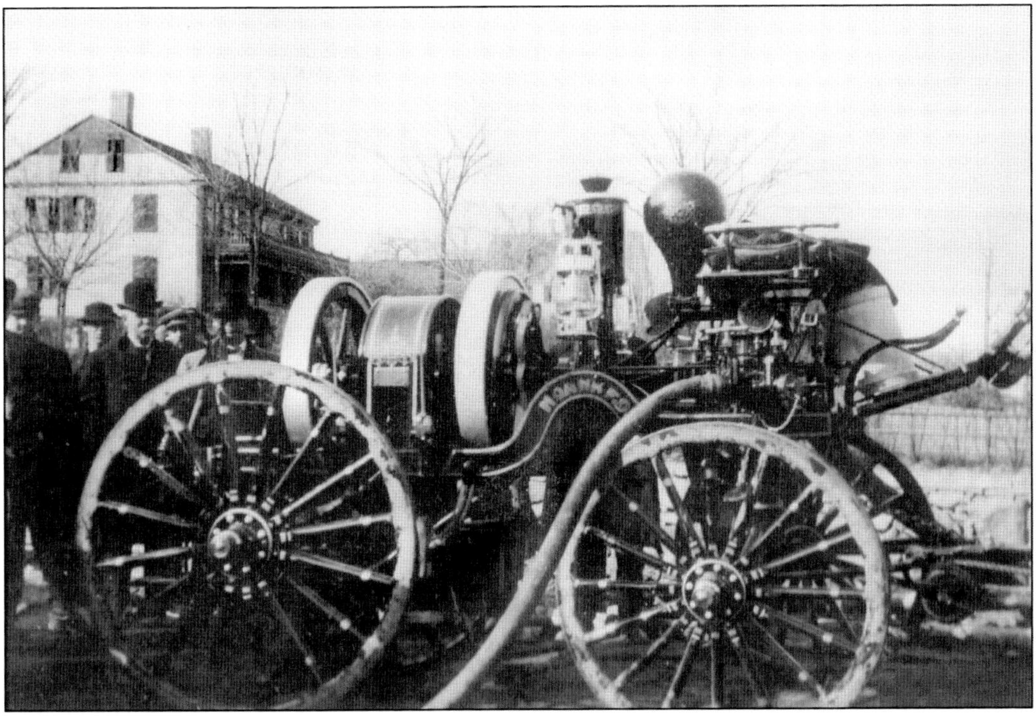

This photograph from the early 1900s shows the Noank Fire Department's horse-drawn, mechanized, gasoline-driven pumper. The picture was taken on Main Street near the town dock in Noank. (Noank Fire Department.)

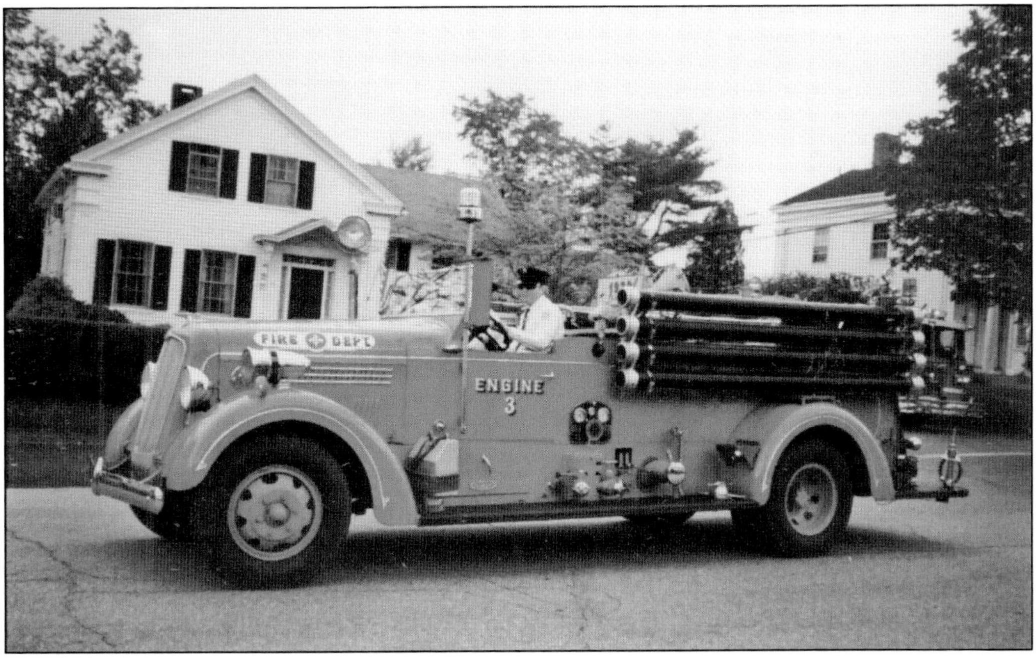

This c. 1980 photograph shows the Noank Fire Department's Engine No. 3, a 1939 Seagrave V-12 engine pumper truck. It is being operated by volunteer firefighter Al Beck during the annual Memorial Day parade along Main Street in Noank. (Noank Fire Department.)

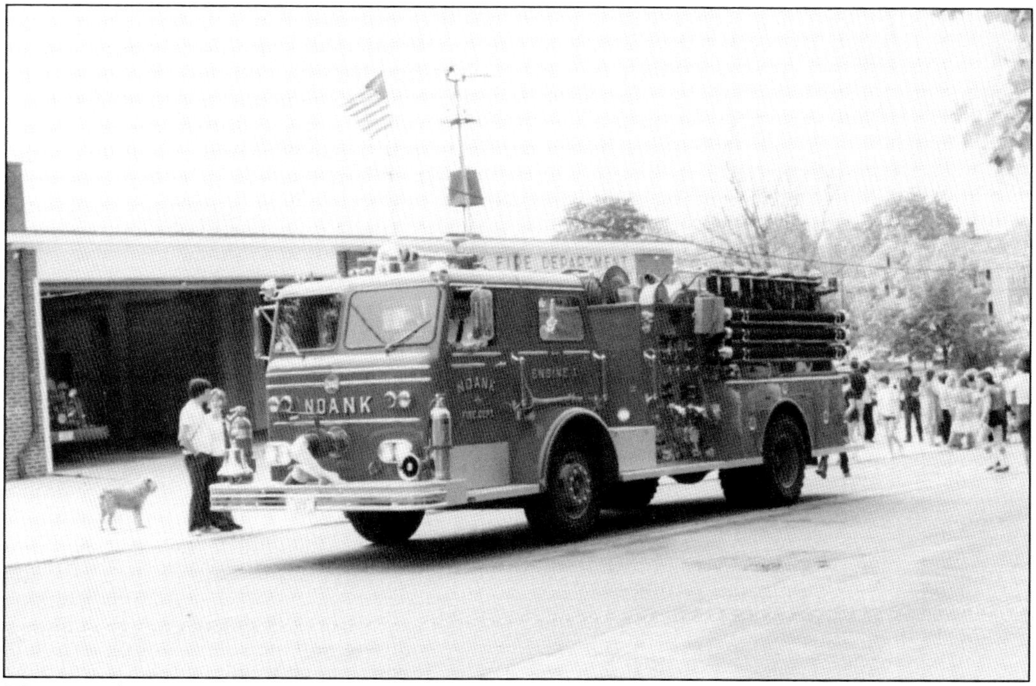

The Noank Fire Department's Engine No. 1, a 1968 Maxim 1,000-gallon-per-minute pumper truck, is pictured in front of the current firehouse on Ward Street prior to a Memorial Day parade. (Noank Fire Department.)

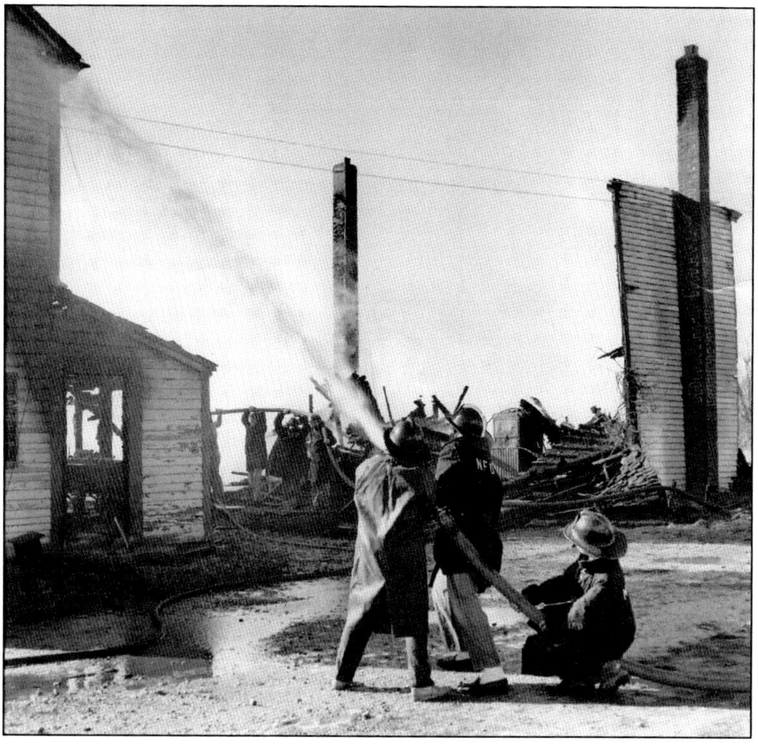

A group of unidentified Noank volunteer firefighters is shown fighting a house fire on Haley Farm on November 11, 1960. The Noank Fire Department responded to assist the Poquonnock Bridge Fire Department in extinguishing this fire. (Noank Fire Department.)

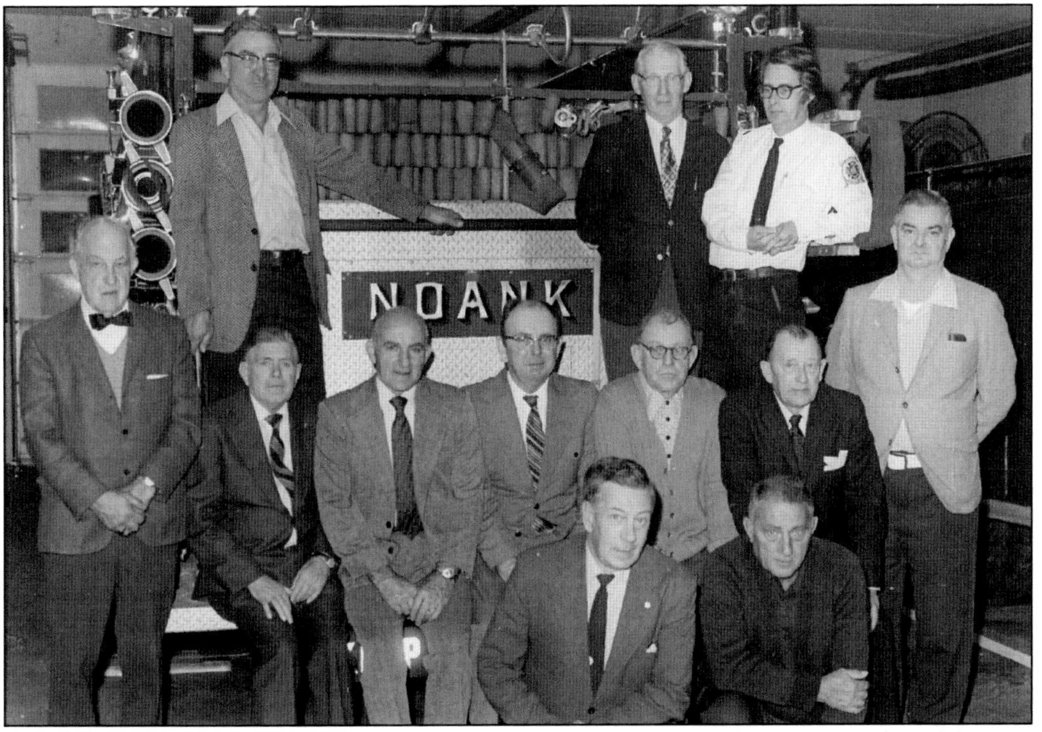

This photograph was taken during the Noank Fire Department's Old-Timers Night celebration in 1974. Pictured on the back of the department's 1968 Maxim pumper truck are, from left to right, (first row) Charlie Halligan and Larry Bunk; (second row) Walter Hold, Edmond Elis, Carlo Bracci, Duncan Carson, Leroy Hodson, Bill Thompson, and George Spader; (third row) Frank Socha, Robert Whittaker, and John Jenssen. (Noank Fire Department.)

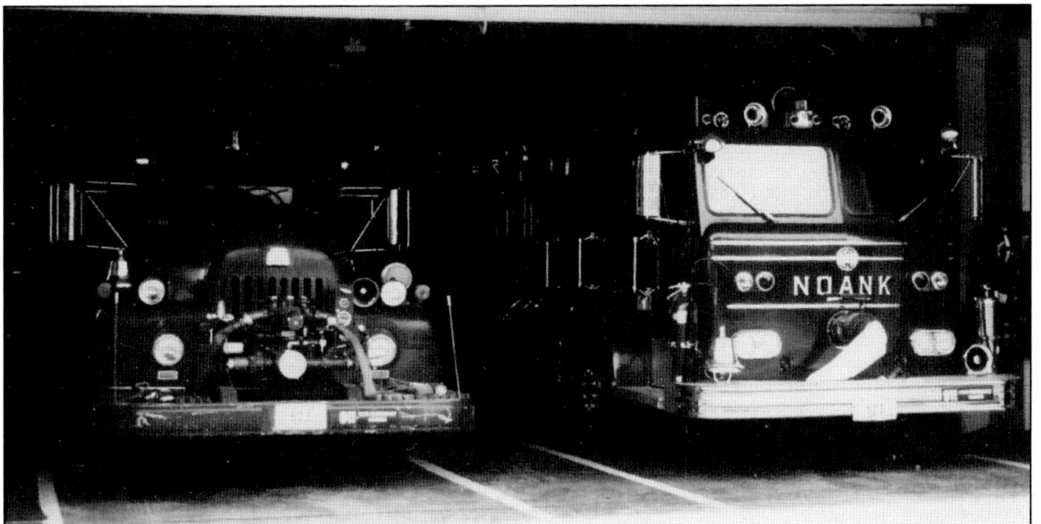

This c. 1970 photograph shows the Noank Fire Department's fire truck parked inside the Ward Street fire station. The vehicle at left is a c. 1949 International front-end pumper that was converted from a 500- to a 750-gallon-per-minute pumper. The truck on the right is a 1968 Maxim 1,000-gallon-per-minute pumper, which was purchased new. (Noank Fire Department.)

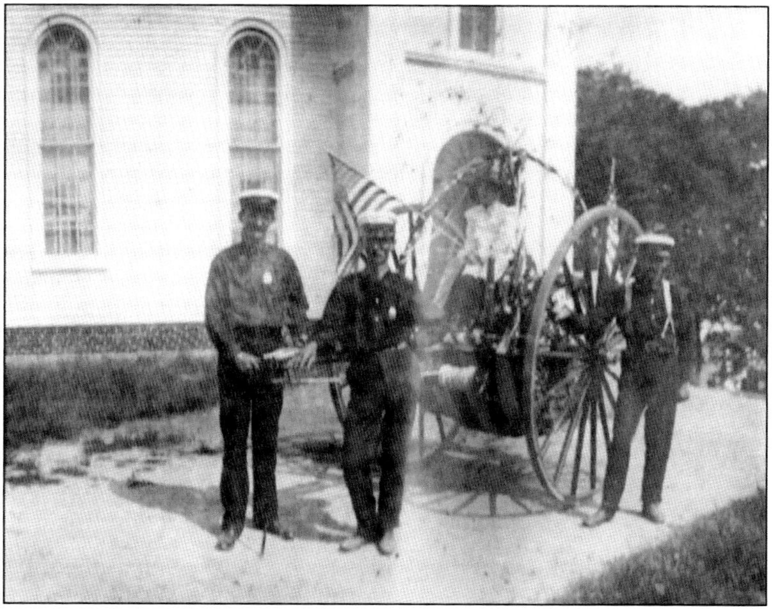

In this c. 1900 photograph, taken in front of the Noank Baptist Church on Main Street, the Noank Fire Department's hose reel apparatus is proudly being displayed by three Noank volunteer firefighters. The man on the left is Hiram Latham, and the child on the top of the reel is Everett Latham; the other two men are unidentified. (Noank Fire Department.)

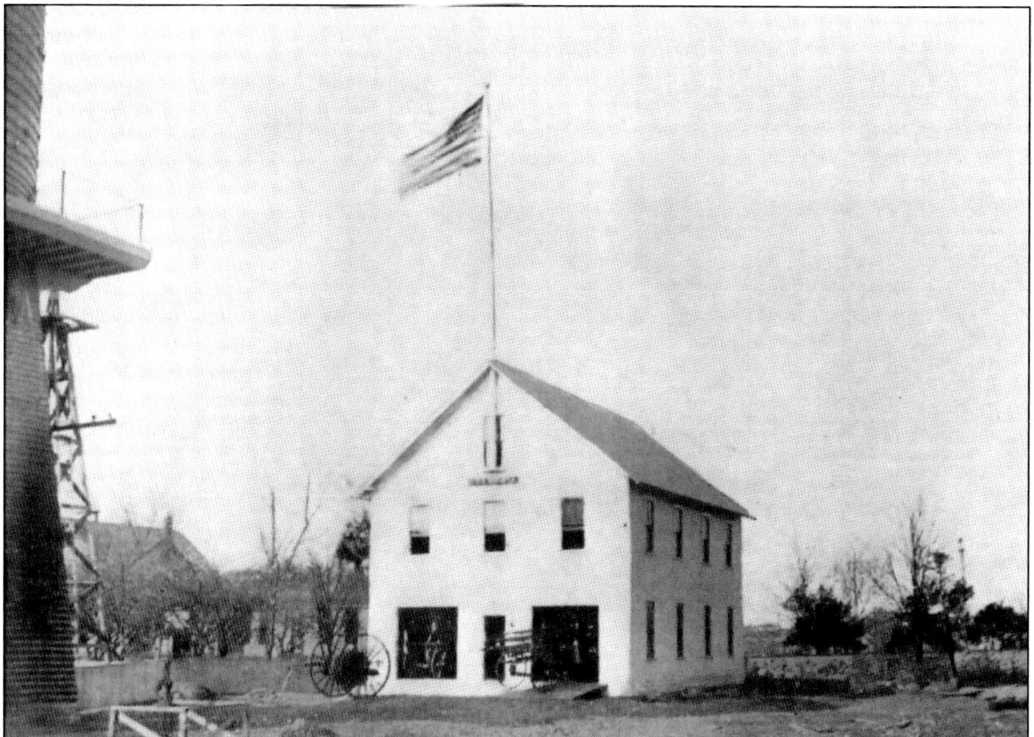

The first Noank firehouse was located on Cedar Street. Several of Noank Fire Department's early horse-drawn firefighting apparatus are shown in this image. Pictured outside is a hose reel. In the left bay is a mechanized gasoline-driven pumper, and in the right bay is a ladder wagon. A large wooden water tower is visible on the far left side of this photograph. The firefighting equipment and water tower were frequently used to extinguish fires at the Palmer shipyard. (Noank Fire Department.)

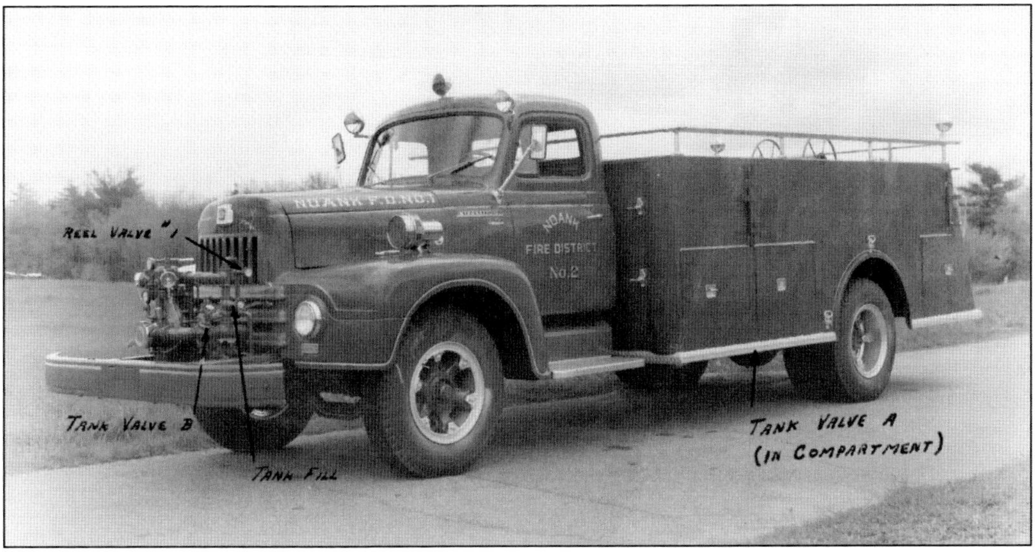

This 1949 photograph shows the Noank Fire Department's newly purchased International 1,000-gallon-per-minute pumper truck. It was designated as Engine No. 2 for the department. (Noank Fire Department.)

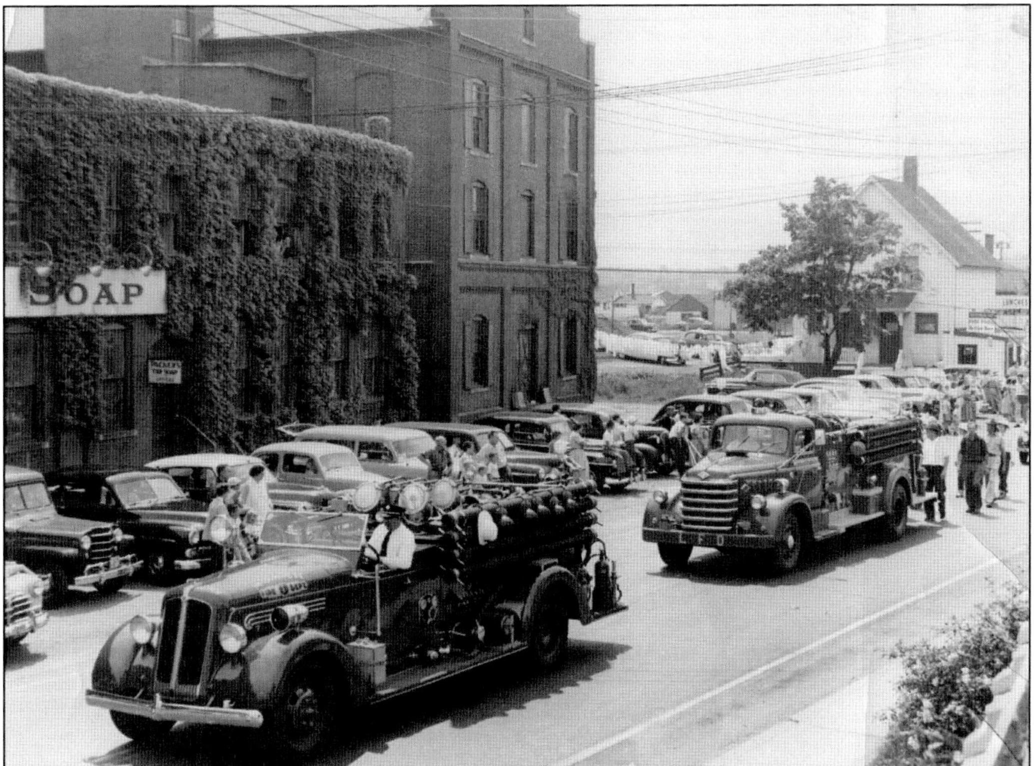

The Noank Fire Department's 1939 Seagraves pumper truck is shown participating in a parade in Mystic in the early 1950s. Volunteer Raymond Coon is operating the vehicle as it passes in front of the Packer's Tar Soap building on Roosevelt Street. (Noank Fire Department.)

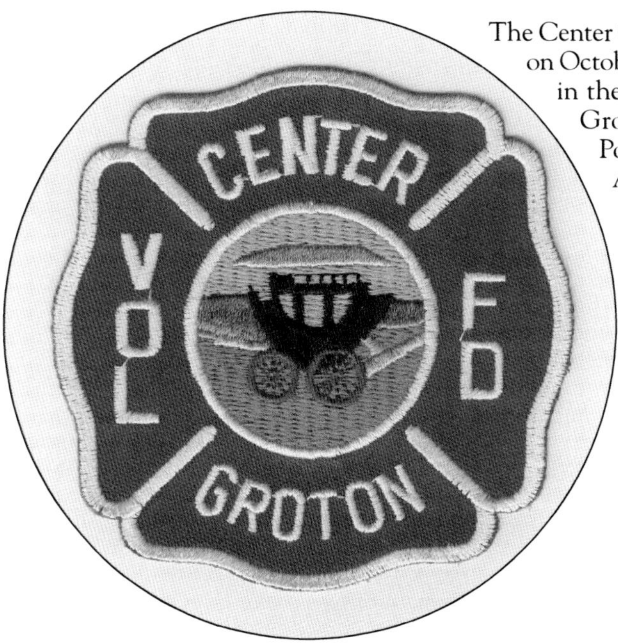

The Center Groton Fire Department was organized on October 6, 1946. Prior to that, fire protection in the area was provided by the Borough of Groton Fire Department and, later, the Poquonnock Bridge Fire Department. A 1928 Chrysler sedan—which was converted to a pickup truck with a 100-gallon tank to supply pack tanks for brushfires—was used as the company's first fire truck. Today, the all-volunteer company maintains a firehouse on Candlewood Road and is equipped with modern firefighting apparatuses. (Center Groton Fire Department.)

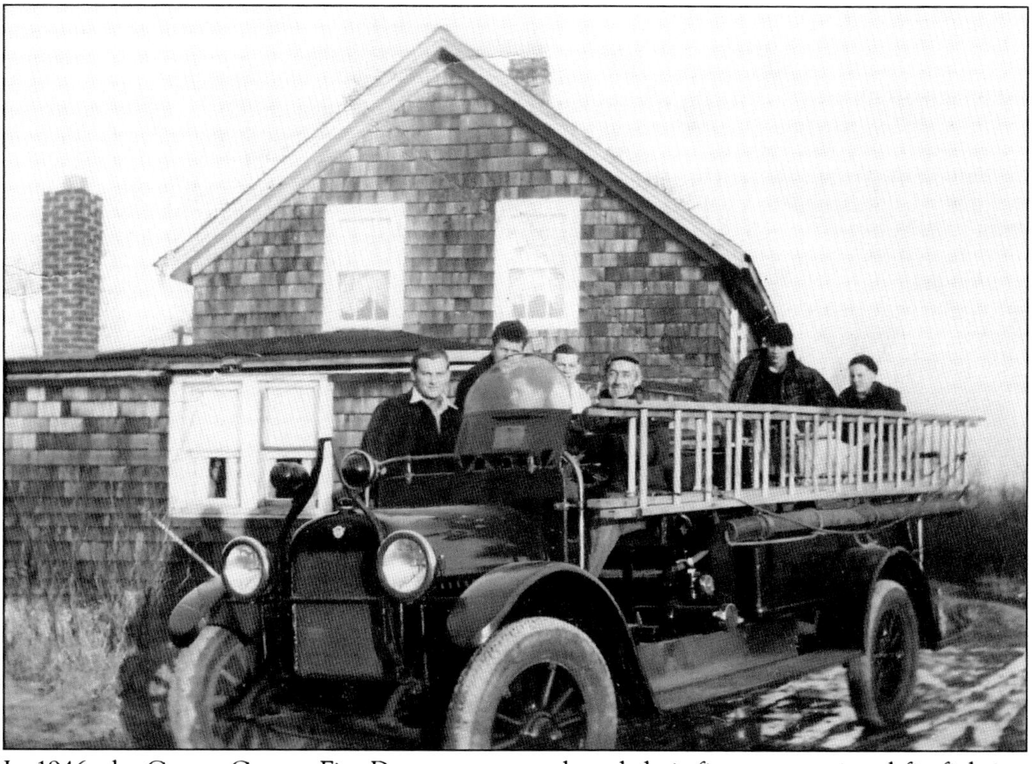

In 1946, the Center Groton Fire Department purchased their first conventional firefighting apparatus—a used 1920 REO pumper truck. The original asking price for the truck was $125, but after some good old Yankee negotiations and consuming four six-packs of beer with the owner, the company purchased the vehicle for $40. Here, unidentified Center Groton Fire Department volunteers proudly display the vehicle in January 1947. (Center Groton Fire Department.)

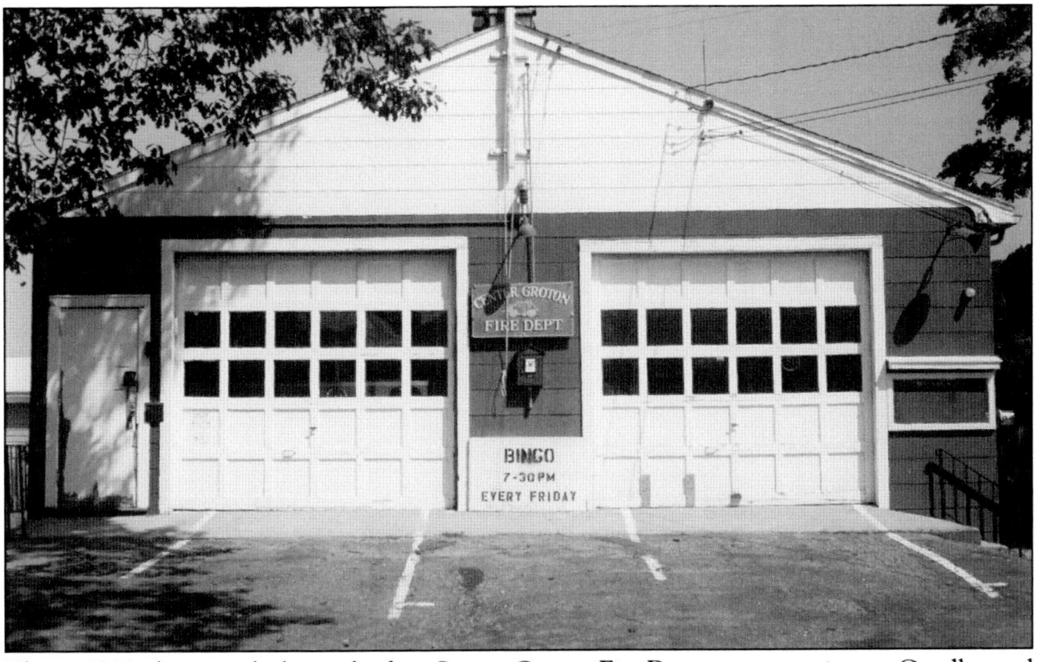

This c. 1980 photograph shows the first Center Groton Fire Department station on Candlewood Road, located next to their current facility. Ground breaking for this building took place in September 1947, and it has been said that the steel beams and lumber from the old highway bridge in Saybrook were used in constructing the fire station's flooring. (Center Groton Fire Department.)

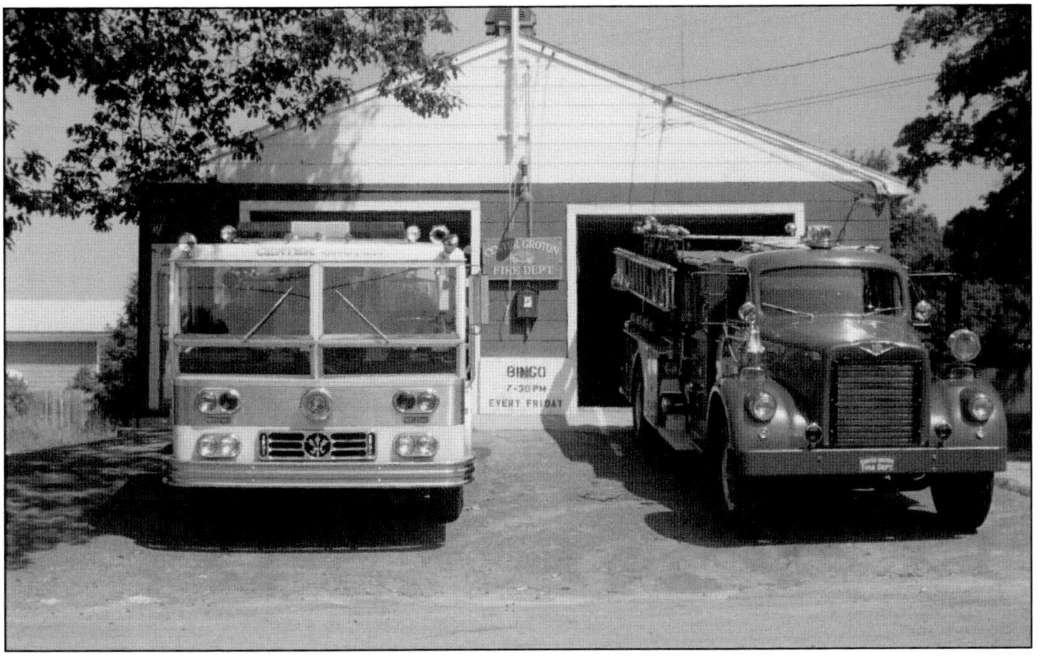

The firefighting apparatuses of the Center Groton Fire Department are pictured in front of the company's station in the late 1970s. At left is a 1974 Ward LaFrance 1,500-gallon-per-minute pumper, and at right is a c. 1950 International 1,000-gallon-per-minute tanker. (Center Groton Fire Department.)

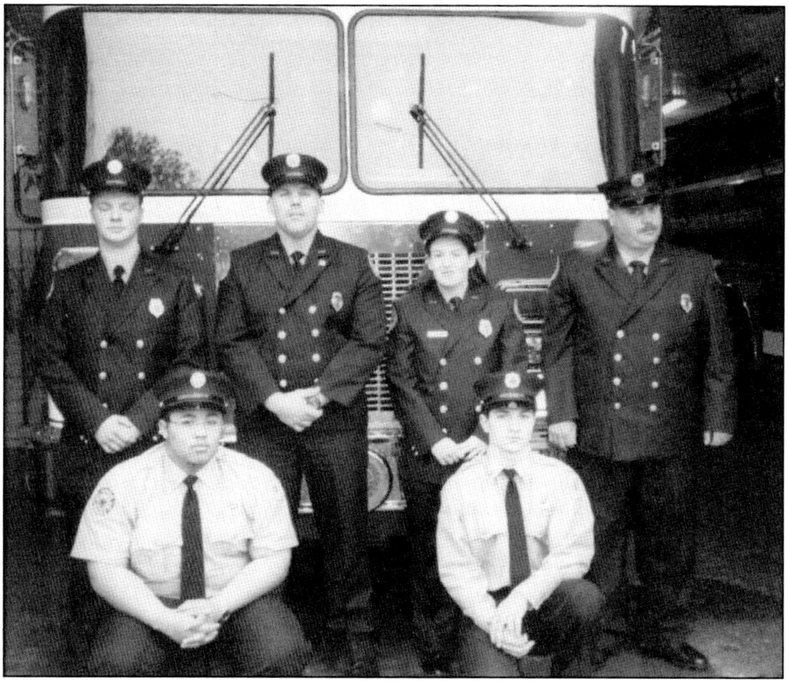

Volunteers with the Center Groton Fire Department posed for this photograph at their station on Candlewood Road. From left to right are (first row) Rasheen Harris and Tony Mancini; (second row) Nick Holiday, John Gordon, Jill Roberts, and Marvin Burkhalter. (Center Groton Fire Department.)

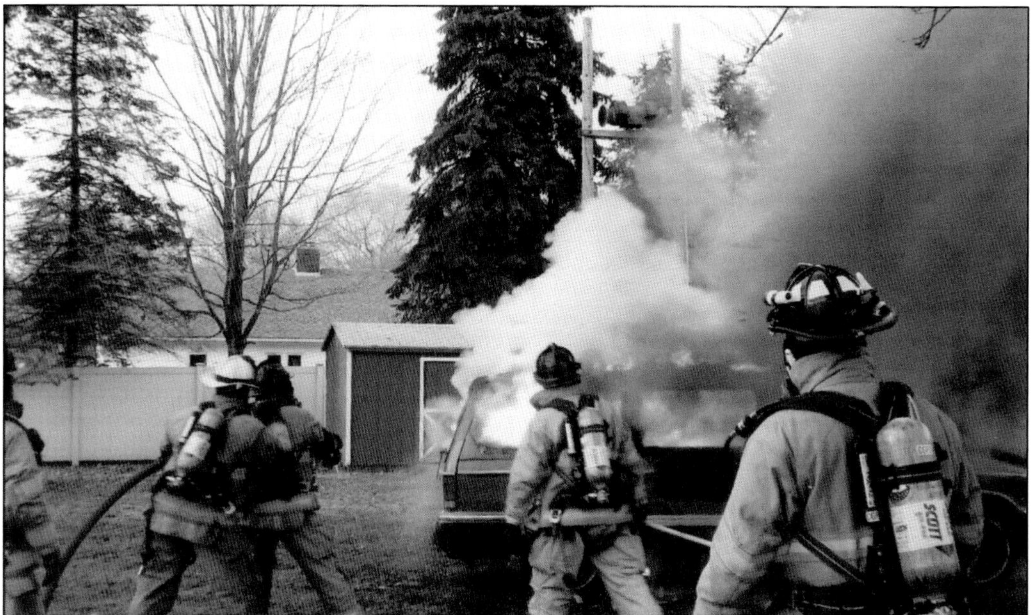

Several unknown volunteer firefighters from the Center Groton Fire Department are shown practicing proper approach techniques while fighting a vehicle fire. Like all other departments, the Center Groton Fire Department conducts training classes throughout the year to sharpen and refresh the firefighting skills of their volunteers. (Center Groton Fire Department.)

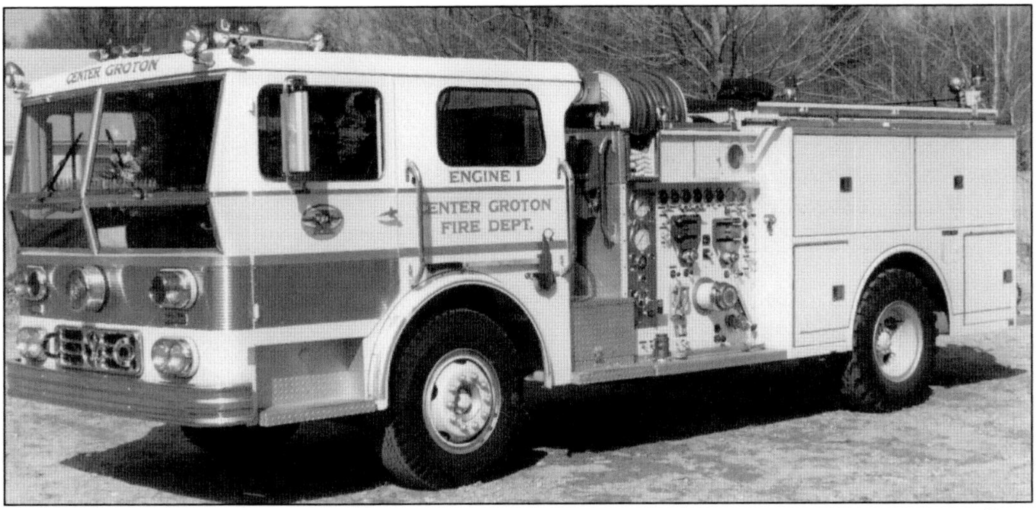

This is the Center Groton Fire Department's Engine No. 1, a 1974 Ward LaFrance 1,500-gallon-per-minute pumper, which was purchased from Farrell, Pennsylvania. When it arrived, the truck was chrome yellow. Members of the company later repainted it red with a white roof to match the department's other apparatus. (Center Groton Fire Department.)

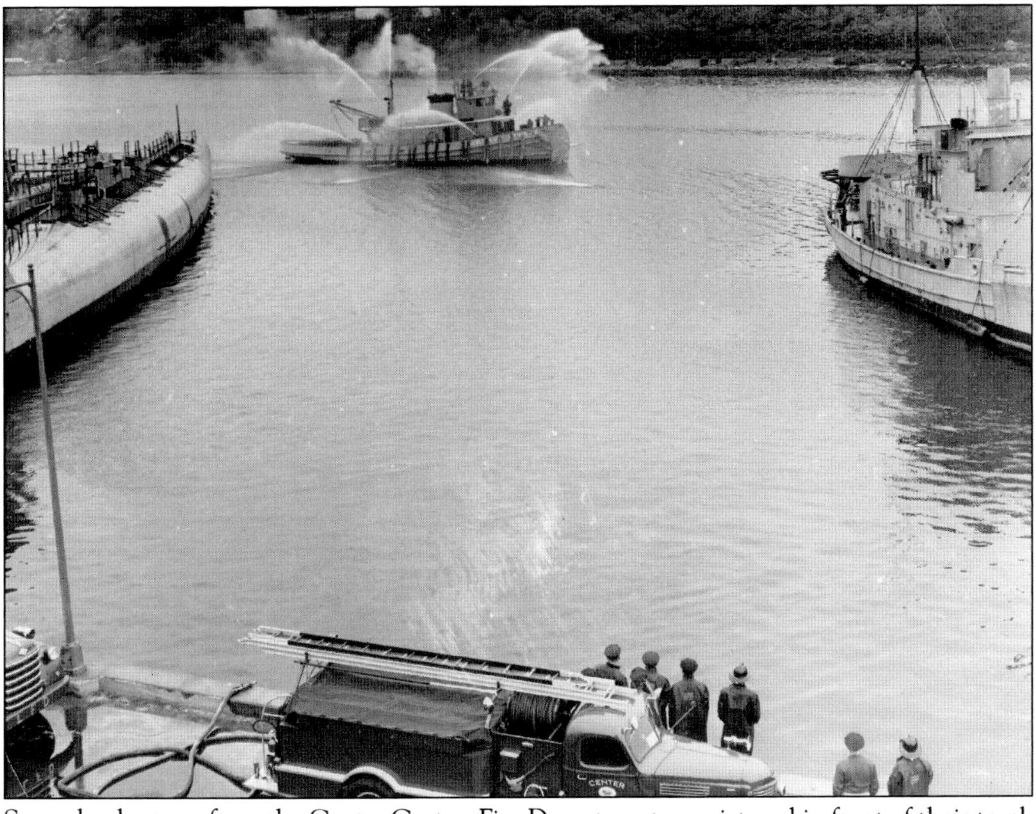

Several volunteers from the Center Groton Fire Department are pictured in front of their truck on a pier at the Naval Submarine Base in Groton during a major civil defense drill in the late 1950s. More than 100 fire departments from throughout the state participated in the "Piggy Back" drill held on May 20, 1957. (Pioneer Hose Company.)

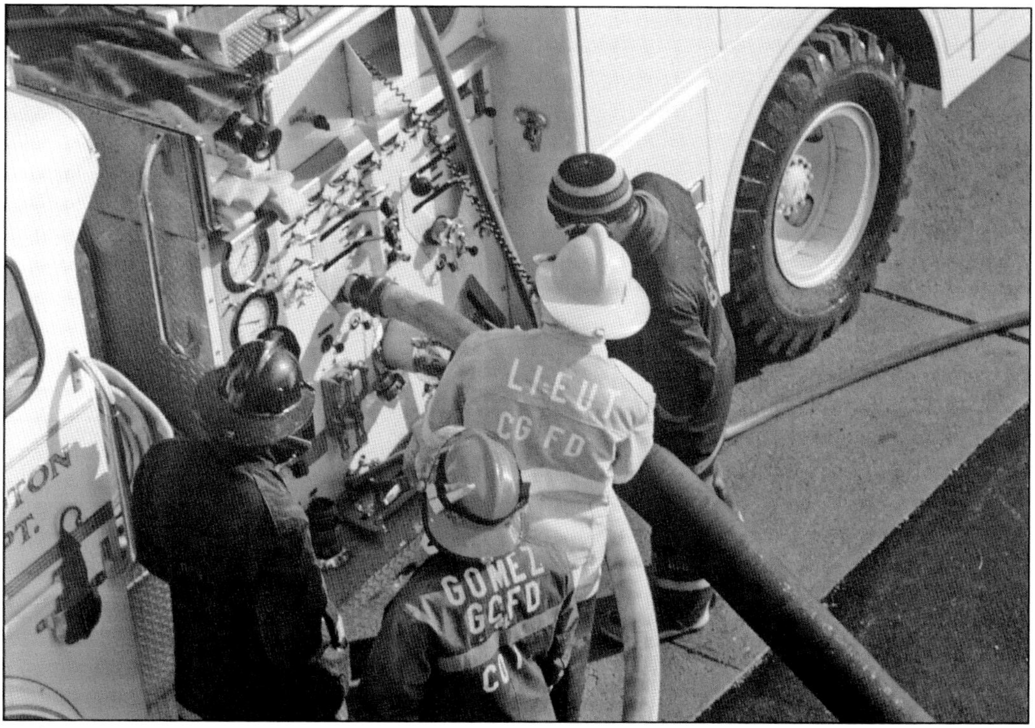

In this c. 1980 image, firefighters from the Center Groton Fire Department and the City of Groton Fire Department conduct a joint training exercise in drafting water from the Washington Park pond using the Center Groton department's pumper truck. (Center Groton Fire Department.)

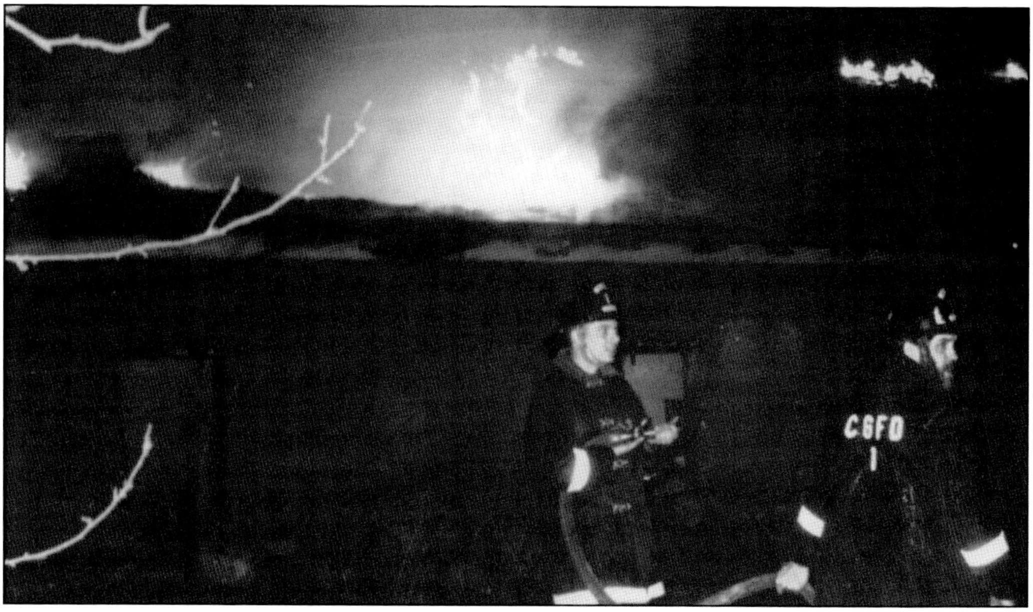

Two unidentified volunteer firefighters from the Center Groton Fire Department are shown assisting with a structural fire at the intersection of Routes 117 and 184 in Groton in November 1973. Their assistance was being provided as part of the mutual aid agreement among all local fire departments. (Center Groton Fire Department.)

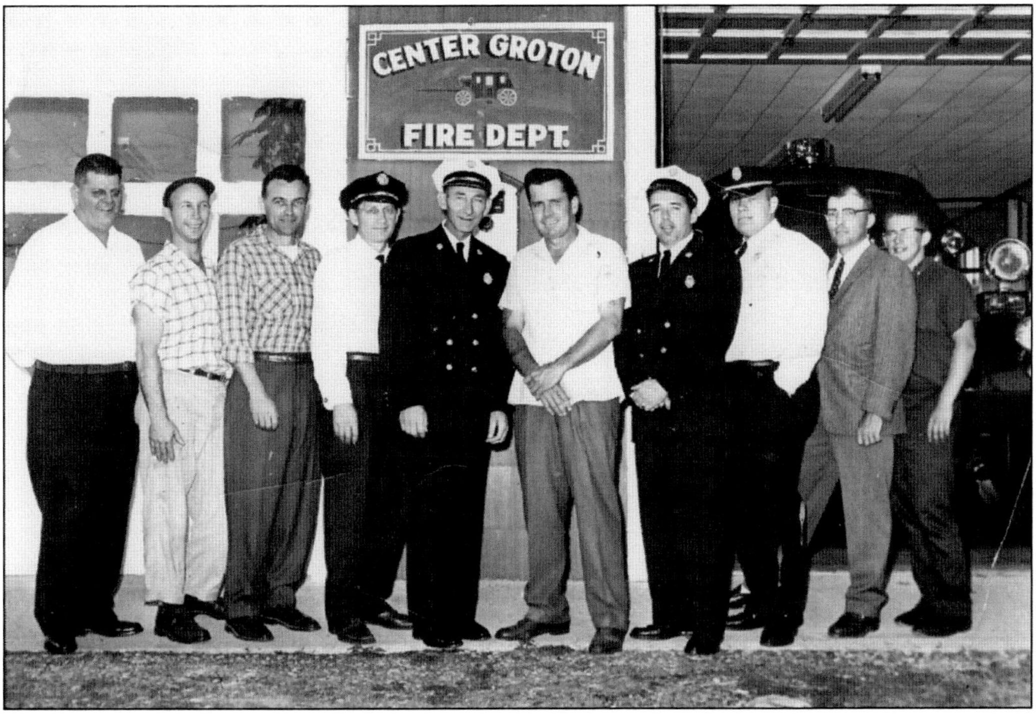

John F. Elliott (fifth from left), the cofounder and first chief of the Center Groton Fire Department, is pictured with fellow firefighters in front of the company's station. Elliott, who died in 1995, served as chief for nine years. (Center Groton Fire Department.)

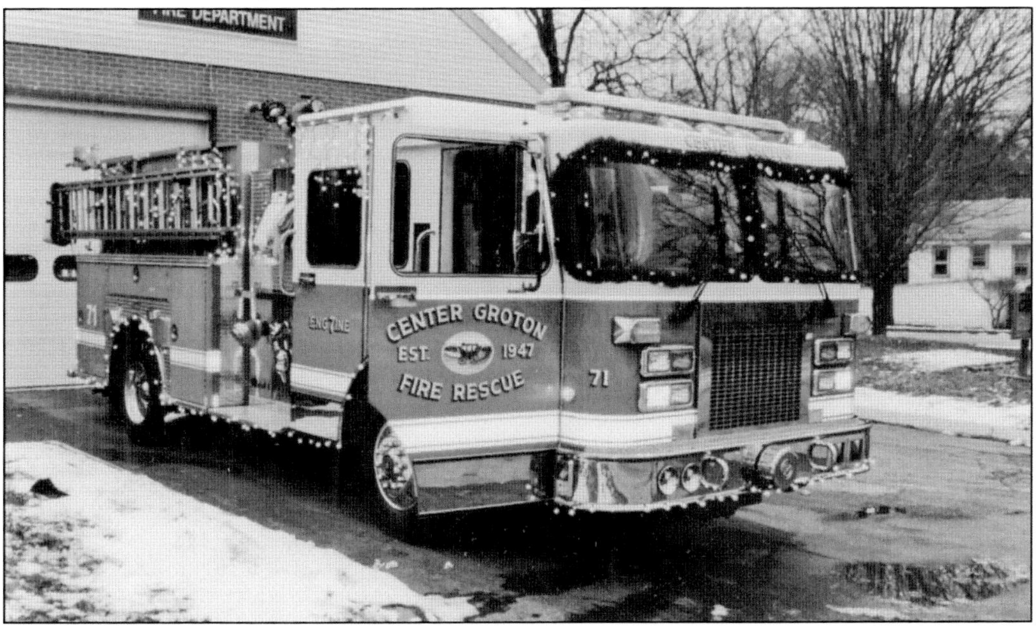

The Center Groton Fire Department's Engine No. 71 is shown decked out in Christmas lights for Groton's annual Holiday Light Parade. Various area fire departments, including Center Groton, have participated in this parade since its inception in the early 2000s. (Center Groton Fire Department.)

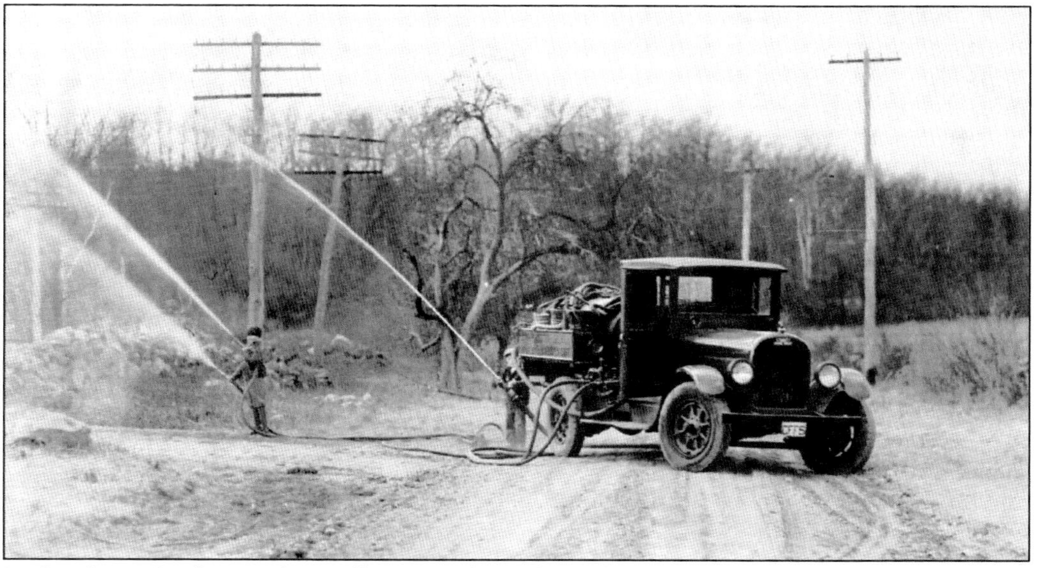

In October 1930, fire warden William D. Alexander and his deputies of the Connecticut Forest Fire Service Groton District built this fire engine with the assistance of O. Pomeroy Robinson and Carl Franzen of Electric Boat. The truck, shown in these c. 1931 images, was equipped with a two-ton chassis, two fire pumps, and a 330-gallon water tank to be used to protect the forested areas in Center Groton and parts of Ledyard. Because the forest fire service had no interest in providing protection to anything other than the forest area in the district, fire protection was provided to the populated area of Center Groton by the Borough of Groton Fire Department until this responsibility was assumed by the Poquonnock Bridge Fire Department. In the fall of 1946, residents of the Center Groton area organized their own fire department. (Both, Iva Alexander Arpin.)

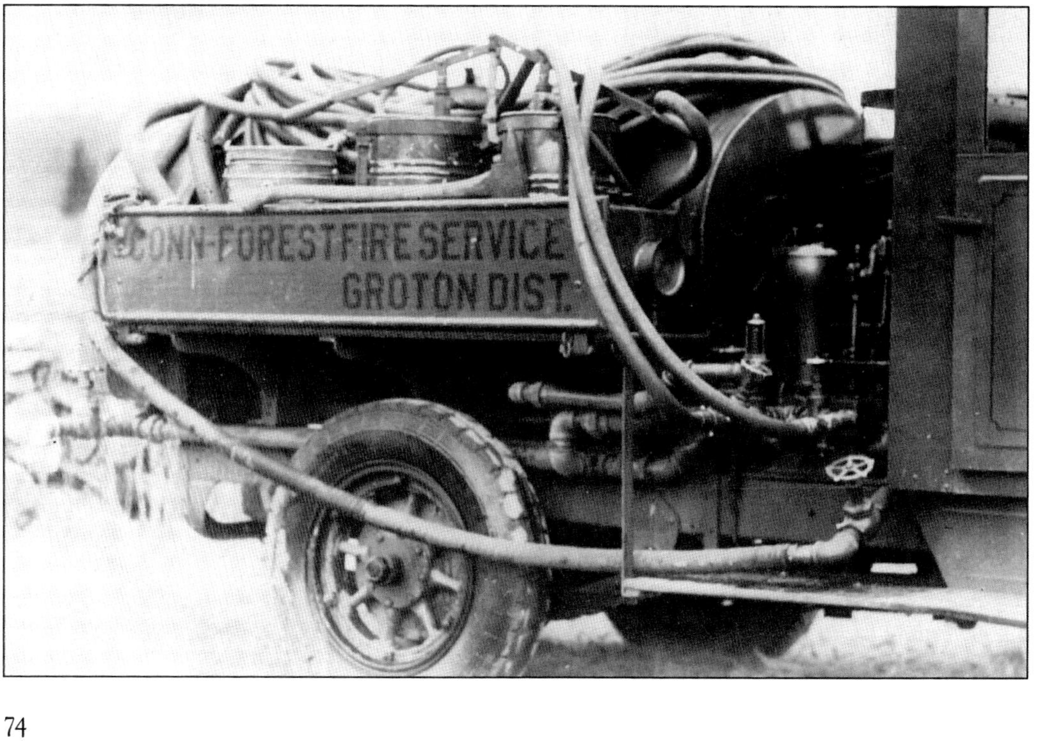

On June 24, 1951, the Groton Long Point Volunteer Fire Department, Inc., was officially established. The Groton Long Point Association had appropriated $20,000 to purchase the company's first fire engine, a 1949 American LaFrance 500-gallon-per-minute pumper on a Ford chassis. Prior to the company's incorporation, fire protection at the Point was provided by the Noank Fire Department, and volunteer firefighters would use a 1922 Buffalo Model T fire truck to fight any fire until the Noank men arrived with their apparatus. Today, the company is still comprised of volunteers, and its equipment is stored in more modern facilities on Atlantic Avenue. (Noank Fire Department.)

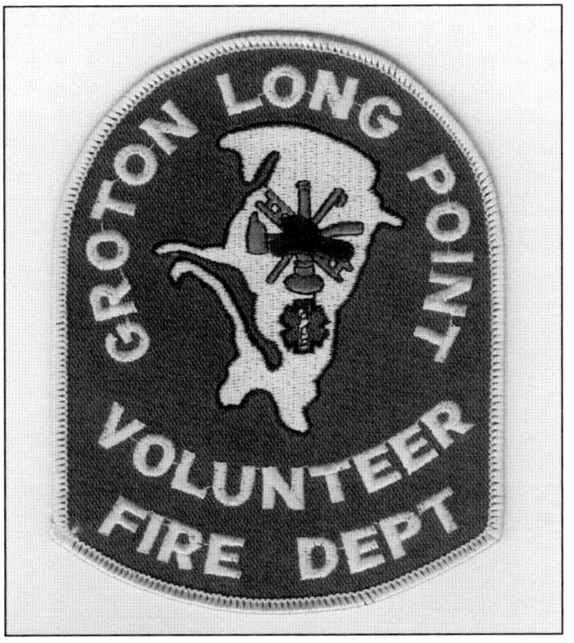

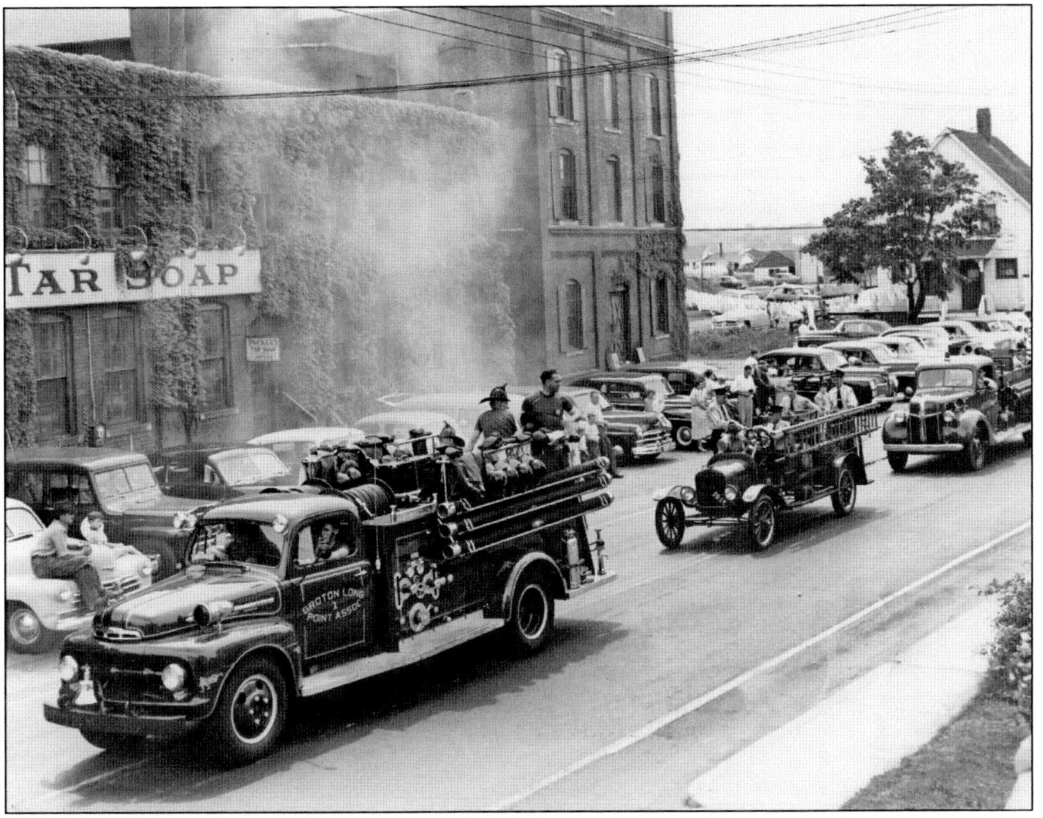

Members of the Groton Long Point Volunteer Fire Company are shown aboard the department's 1949 American LaFrance pumper truck as it passes the Packer's Tar Soap building on Roosevelt Avenue in Mystic during a parade in the early 1950s. (Jim Streeter.)

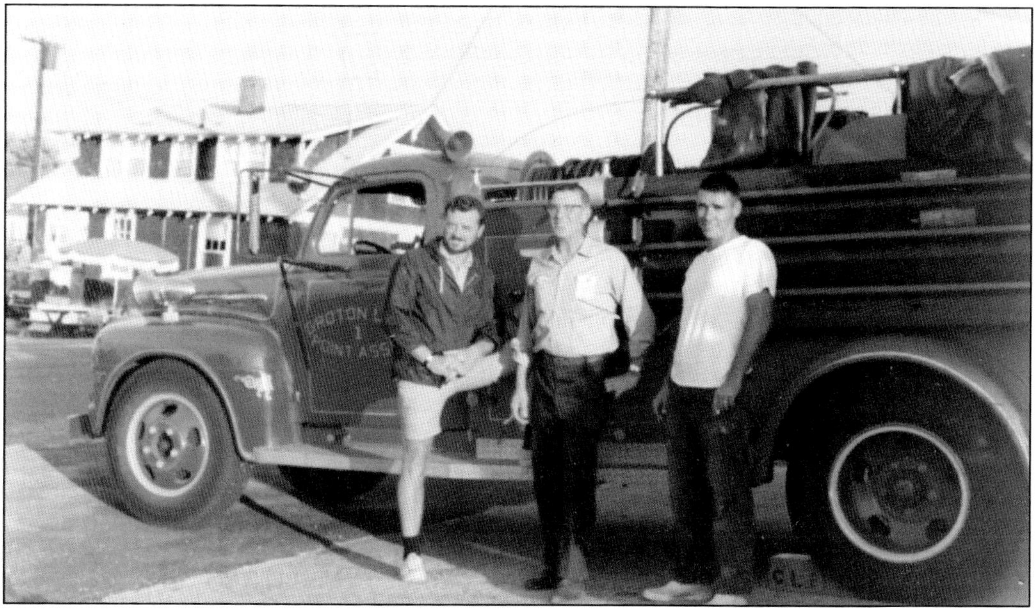

Members of the Groton Long Point Volunteer Fire Company are pictured in front of the department's 1949 American LaFrance 500-gallon-per-minute pumper truck in September 1968. From left to right are Al Russo, George Bigbee, and Dave Walker. (Groton Long Point Association.)

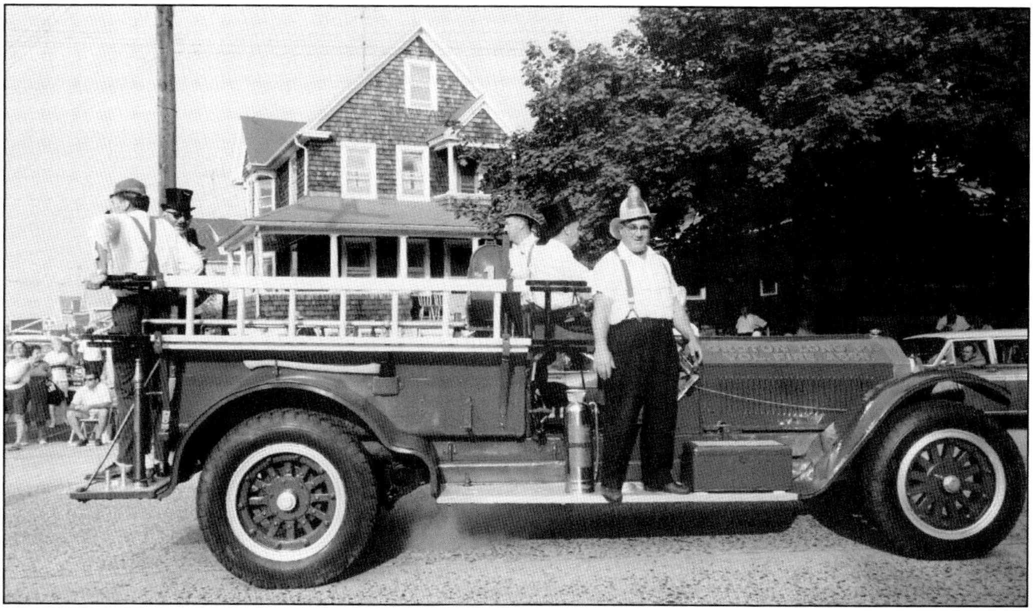

Several volunteer members of the Groton Long Point Volunteer Fire Company proudly display the department's antique fire apparatus, a 1917 American LaFrance truck known as "Alfie," during a parade in New London in 1966. The Groton Long Point Volunteer Fire Company purchased the vehicle from the Watch Hill Fire Department in Rhode Island in 1966. In March 1980, it was sold to an unknown buyer and later found in storage at Seaport Marine in Mystic. In 1987, Seaport Marine donated the vehicle back to the Groton Long Point Volunteer Fire Company. The company has since completely restored the vehicle and continues to display it at various parades throughout New England. (Pioneer Hose Company.)

Two

Military, Industrial, and Other Fire Departments

Groton, Connecticut, is home to the Naval Submarine Base New London, which is the home port for 15 nuclear submarines and the "university" for submarine training. The base comprises 680 acres and provides support facilities and services to the men and women stationed there, as well as their families. The submarine base also provides 2,100 dependent-housing units on an additional 530 acres off base. The average overall daily population at the base exceeds approximately 15,000. Needless to say, the base is a city within itself. A dedicated fire department provides much of the emergency services to the base and its housing facilities.

Two major industrial facilities are also located in Groton. Electric Boat, a General Dynamics company, designs, builds, and repairs nuclear submarines and maintains facilities on 112 acres and currently employs approximately 8,500 workers. It also has a dedicated fire department that provides emergency services on the company's property. Pfizer Inc. maintains its primary research and development laboratories on 160 acres in Groton. Approximately 4,500 employees work in state-of-the-art facilities situated on 2.8 million square feet of acreage. Due to the complexity of the chemical materials used at the company, their specially trained fire department responds to all of the emergencies at this corporate campus.

The Groton–New London Airport, a publicly owned general aviation airport, is also located in Groton. The airport provides facilities for corporate jets as well as multi- and single-engine aircraft. The 489-acre site is also home to the Army National Guard 1109th Theater Aviation Sustainment Maintenance Group (TASMG), which repairs and maintains military helicopters. This airport maintains a fire/rescue and maintenance department to respond to all emergency incidents on their property.

In addition to the above departments, Groton previously had two other facilities that provided firefighting aid. The US Coast Guard maintained a large training school at Avery Point, and the Hess Oil Corporation operated an oil/diesel/kerosene wholesale distribution terminal near Pfizer. Both facilities maintained firefighting apparatus to control small fires until the City of Groton Fire Department could respond to the scene.

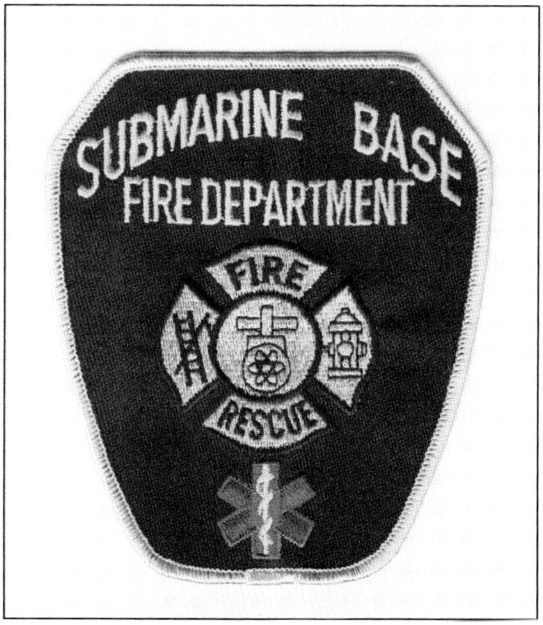

The Submarine Base Fire Department was organized in 1942. It is believed that military personnel augmented the career staff in the beginning. As the base has grown, so has the fire department. They now have two shifts of 20 firefighters manning up-to-date fire apparatus. In addition to typical services, the Submarine Base Fire Department started a Hazardous Materials Team in 1987 to handle incidents involving hazardous materials. They also initiated a Rapid Intervention Team that is trained to rescue firefighters who become trapped while fighting a fire. They ensure readiness at the shore, protecting the fleet, fighter, and family for the submarine base, and they work closely with the community, taking pride in "protecting those who defend America." (Submarine Base New London Fire Department.)

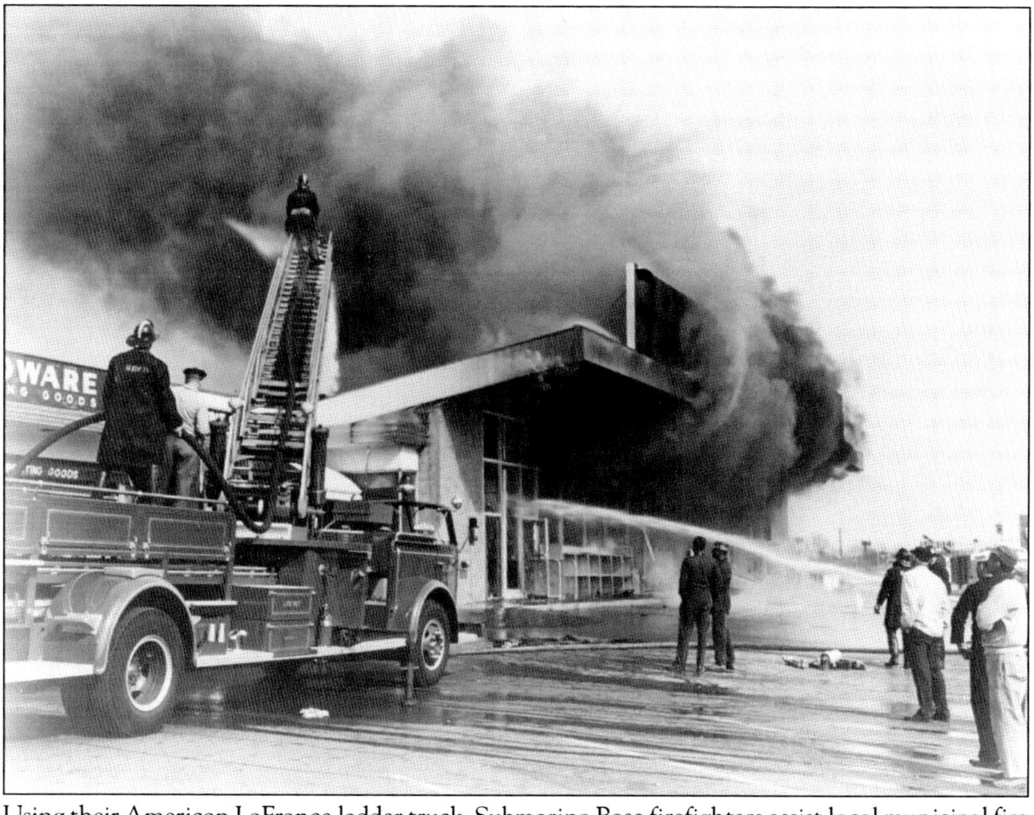

Using their American LaFrance ladder truck, Submarine Base firefighters assist local municipal fire departments in extinguishing a major fire that destroyed the First National Food Stores building in the Groton Shopping Plaza on April 29, 1963. One of the firemen is on the end of the extended ladder, in the billowing smoke, applying water to the roof of the building. (Jim Streeter.)

Submarine Base Fire Department assistant chief Kenneth Jeffrey, a 20-year veteran of the department, suffered a heart attack while on duty at the station on Christmas Day 2003 and subsequently died on New Year's Eve of that year. His is the only line-of-duty death that has occurred within the Submarine Base Fire Department. (Submarine Base New London Fire Department.)

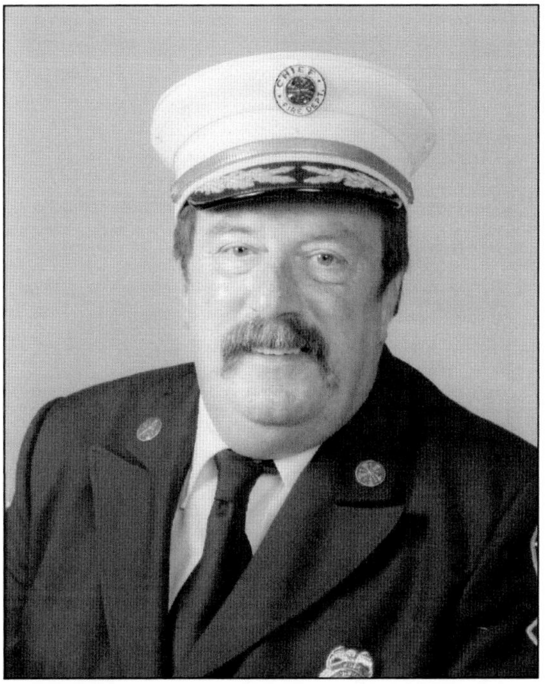

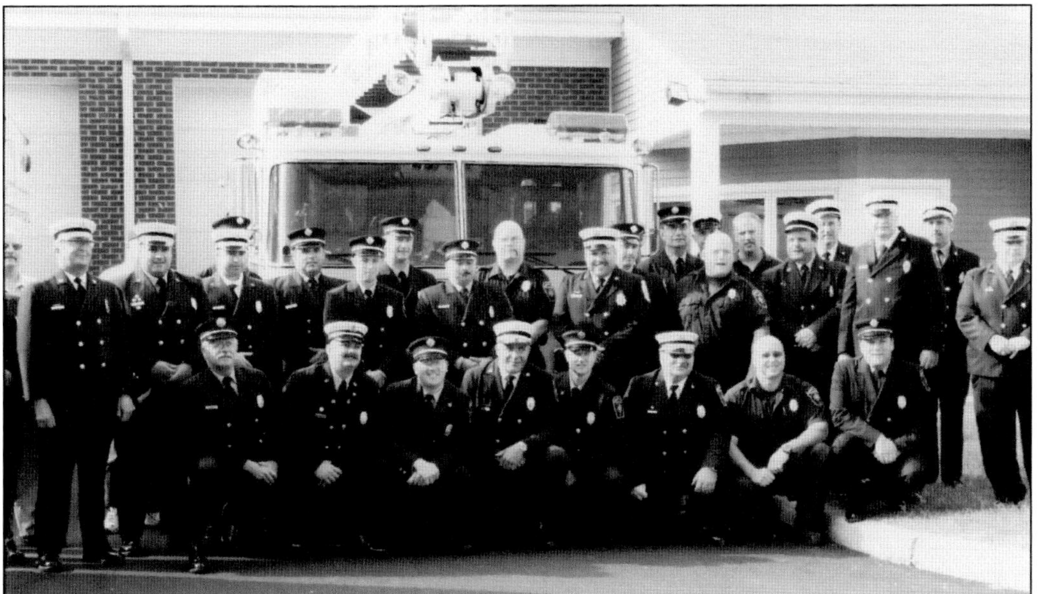

In this May 2008 photograph, the firefighting staff of the Submarine Base Fire Department proudly posed in front of the fire headquarters on base. From left to right are (first row) John Dwire Sr., Patrick O'Brien, Chris Whipple, Doug Say, Robert O'Brien, Jeff King, Robert Ormond, and Robert Ladd; (second row) Dave Steel, Stephen Lougee, Andy Willey, Mike Spinnato, Maurice Remillard, Thomas Clapsadle, Mike Schneider, Robert Kelley, John McDonald, and Les Shull; (third row) Fred Stone, John Dwire Jr., Jeff Post, Peter Woodbury, Scott Morris, Tim Johnson, Keith Andrews, Keith Knudsen, Jay Borcuk, and Anthony Saccone. (Submarine Base New London Fire Department.)

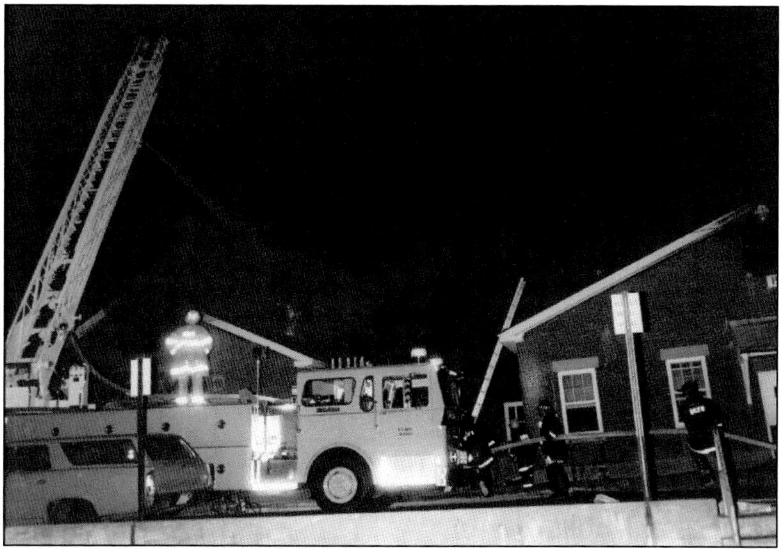

Firefighters are pictured at the scene of a major fire that occurred at a complex containing five adjoining buildings on the Naval Submarine Base New London in Groton on July 13, 1980. The fire caused an estimated $5 million in damage. (Submarine Base New London Fire Department.)

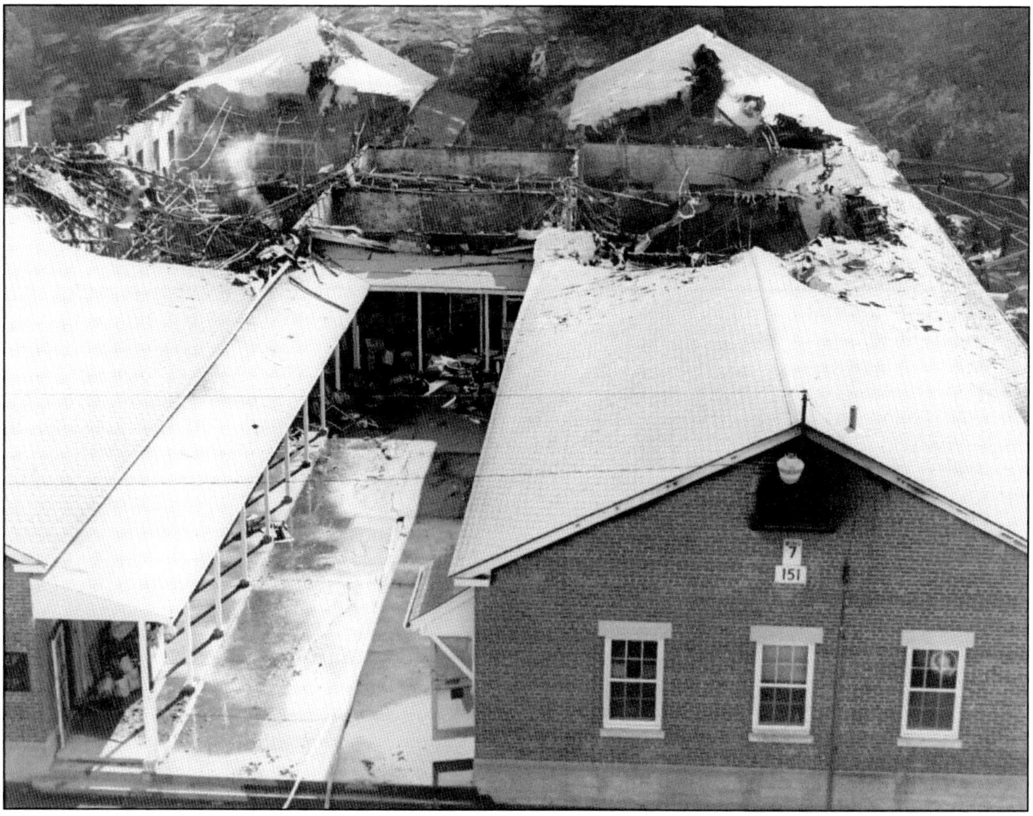

This aerial view shows the extensive damage that resulted from the fire at a five-building Navy Exchange complex on July 13, 1980. Numerous buildings were affected, including the Sub Base Print Shop, the Naval Exchange Thrift Shop, the Bachelors' Enlisted Quarters supply area, a supply operations office, and two women's and children's apparel stores. (Submarine Base New London Fire Department.)

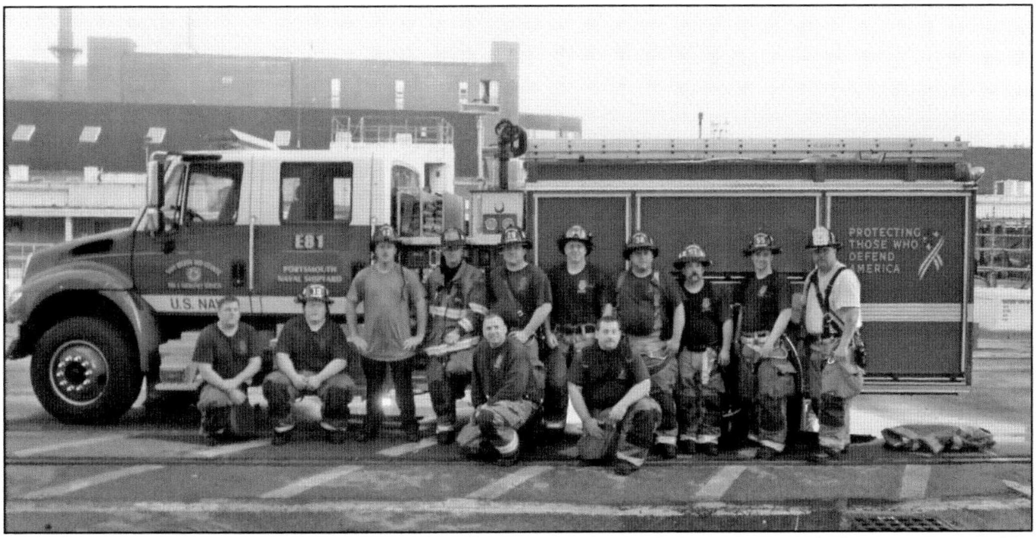

On May 23 and 24, 2012, Submarine Base New London firefighters responded to a catastrophic fire on the nuclear-powered submarine USS *Miami* at the Portsmouth Naval Shipyard in New Hampshire. Pictured here are the personnel who responded. From left to right are (first row) Wager and Gauette; (second row) Ladd, Schneider, Knudsen, Captain Post, MacDonald, Ormond, Dwire, Keaten, Canavan, and Captain Woodbury. The unexpected response to the *Miami* fire caused a significant void in the normal scheduling for the department, and the remaining personnel went the extra mile by working extended hours to ensure continued fire protection at the base. (Submarine Base New London Fire Department.)

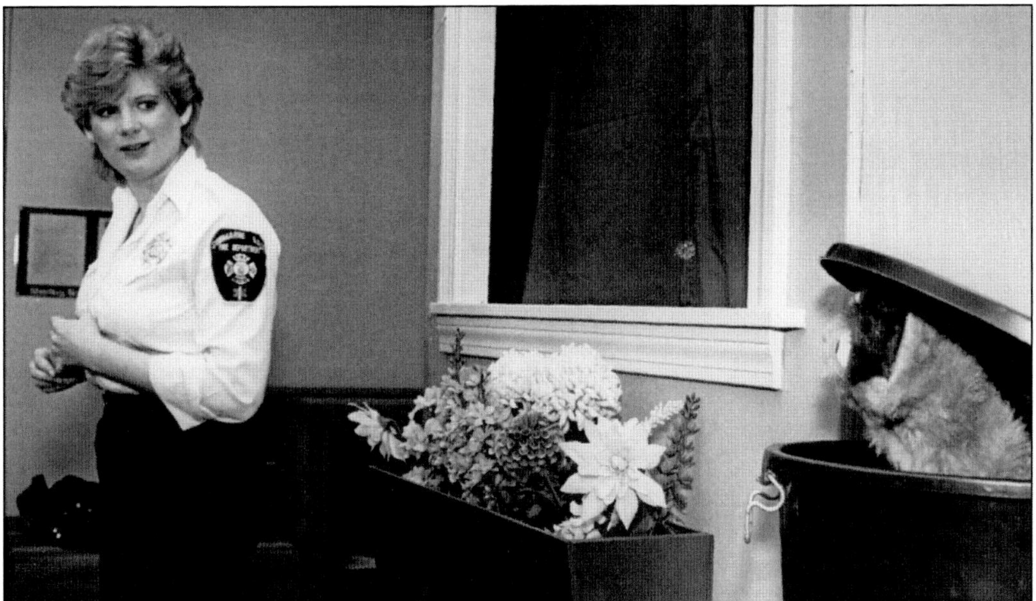

Submarine Base New London fire inspector Lisa Gale is shown having a discussion with Sesame Street character Oscar the Grouch (at far right) at a special fire prevention program for children that was held on the submarine base on April 16, 1985. The Submarine Base Fire Department conducts many fire prevention programs for children of Navy personnel assigned to the base. (Submarine Base New London Fire Department.)

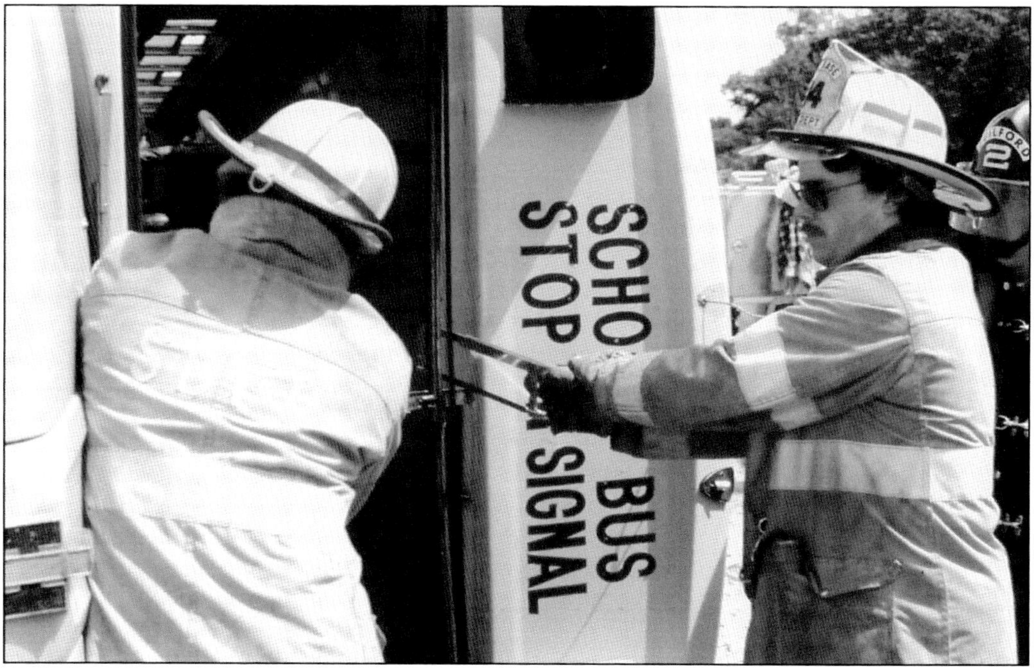

Firefighter John Keating (right) and an unidentified firefighter from the Submarine Base Fire Department participate in Connecticut's first heavy rescue training course in June 1983. This course involved entering a school bus and extricating passengers. Fire departments are constantly seeking training involving various situations that they may someday encounter. (Submarine Base New London Fire Department.)

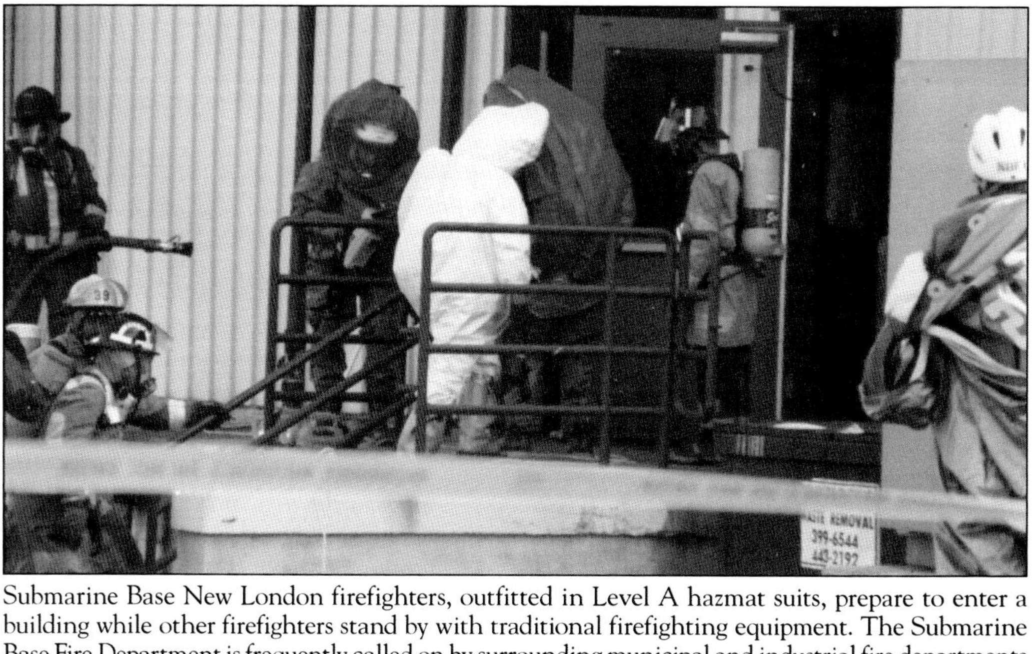

Submarine Base New London firefighters, outfitted in Level A hazmat suits, prepare to enter a building while other firefighters stand by with traditional firefighting equipment. The Submarine Base Fire Department is frequently called on by surrounding municipal and industrial fire departments to assist in hazmat-related incidents because it is equipped with special response equipment and apparatus. (Submarine Base New London Fire Department.)

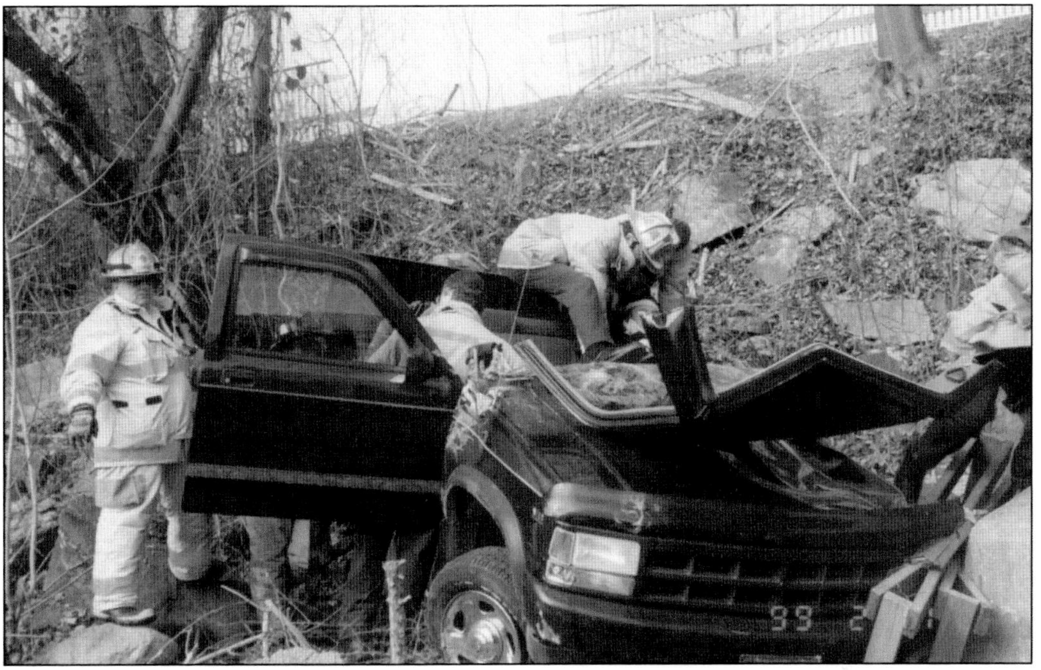

Chief Lester Shull supervises Submarine Base New London firefighters in extricating and providing medical attention to the driver of a pickup truck that had rolled down an embankment after crashing through a fence in February 1999. (Submarine Base New London Fire Department.)

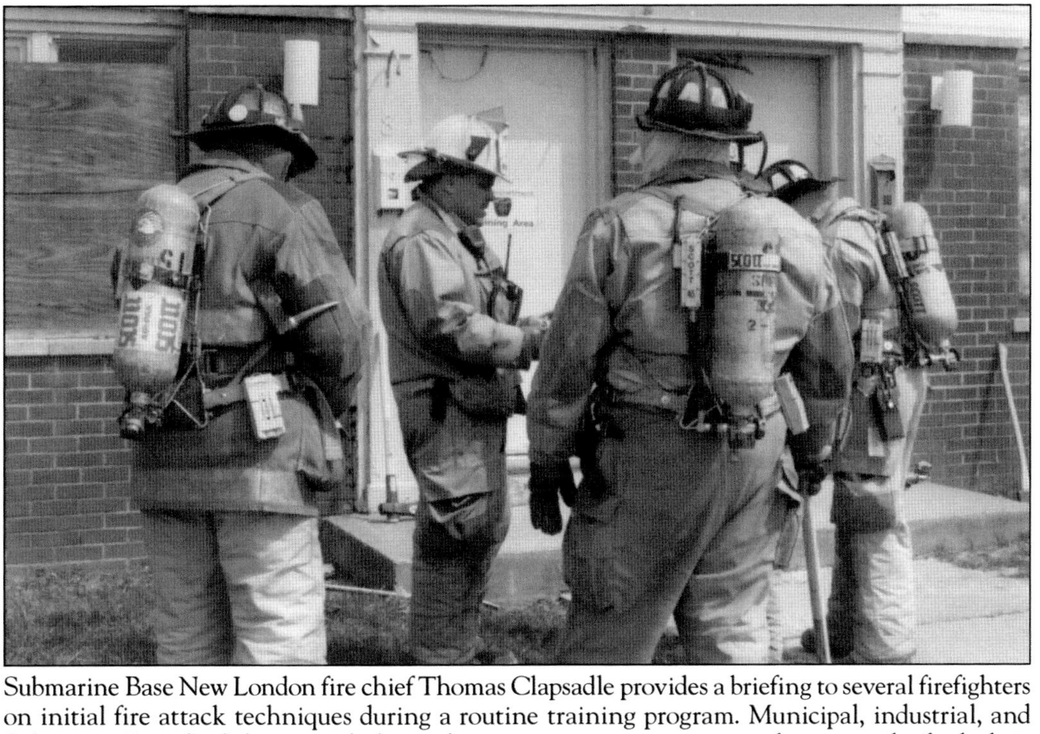

Submarine Base New London fire chief Thomas Clapsadle provides a briefing to several firefighters on initial fire attack techniques during a routine training program. Municipal, industrial, and Submarine Base firefighters regularly conduct joint training exercises to sharpen and refresh their firefighting skills. (Submarine Base New London Fire Department.)

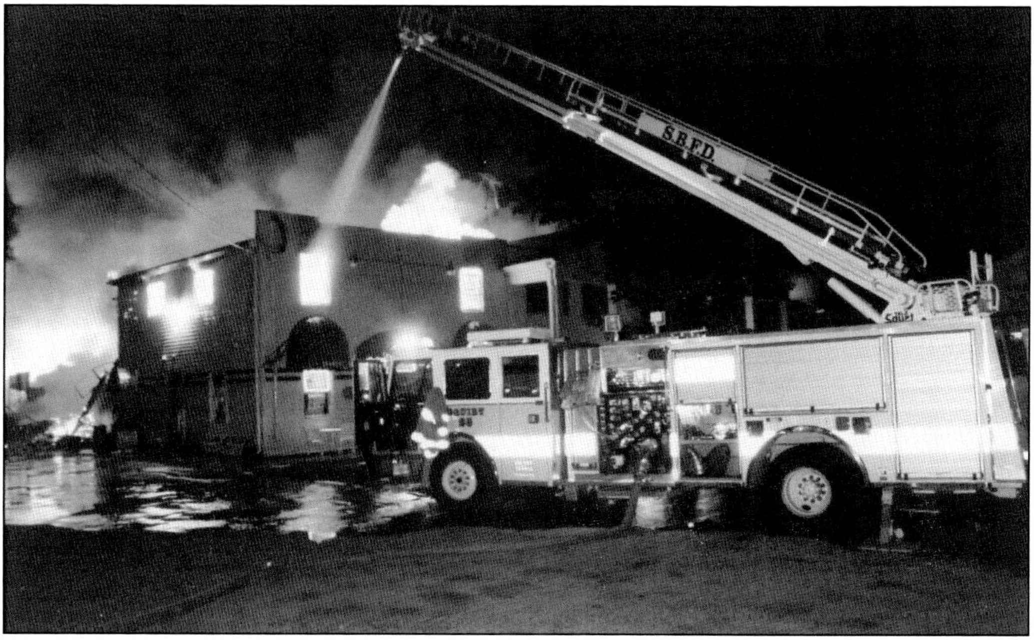

On August 18, 1999, the Submarine Base Fire Department was called to assist local municipal fire departments in fighting a major fire that resulted in the destruction of a large business complex on Route 184 in Groton. The building housed a furniture store, an electronics store, a pizza restaurant, an antique shop, and a guitar shop. (Submarine Base New London Fire Department.)

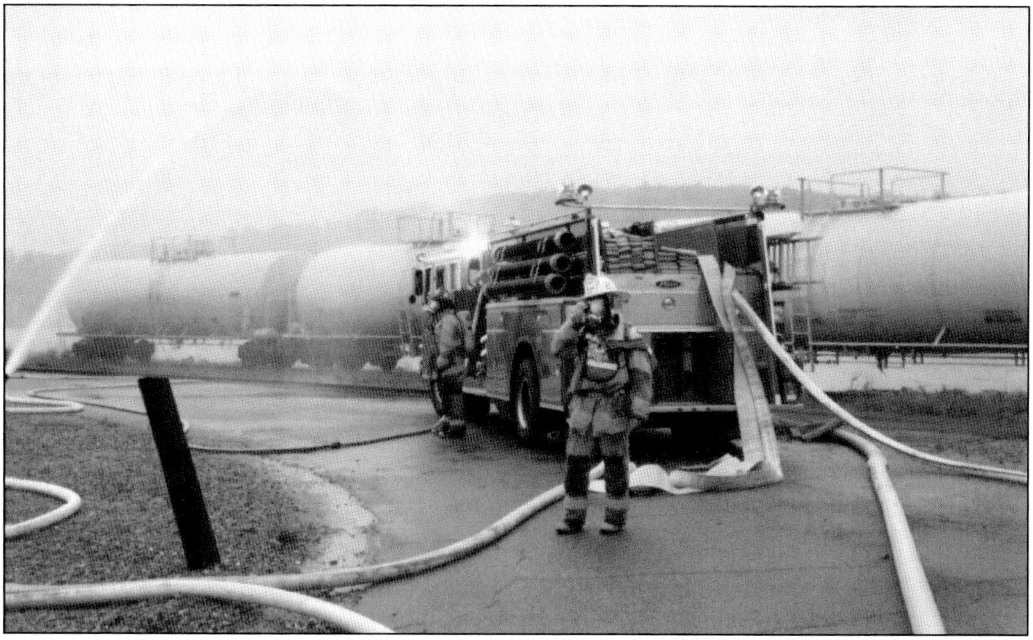

As part of their hazmat training program, Submarine Base New London personnel use a fire hose to spray several railroad chemical tanks to keep them cool and to prevent a rupture or explosion. These training exercises are conducted on a regular basis due to the fact that chemical railcars frequently travel via tracks that run through the property and also due to the proximity of the base to a neighboring chemical company. (Submarine Base New London Fire Department.)

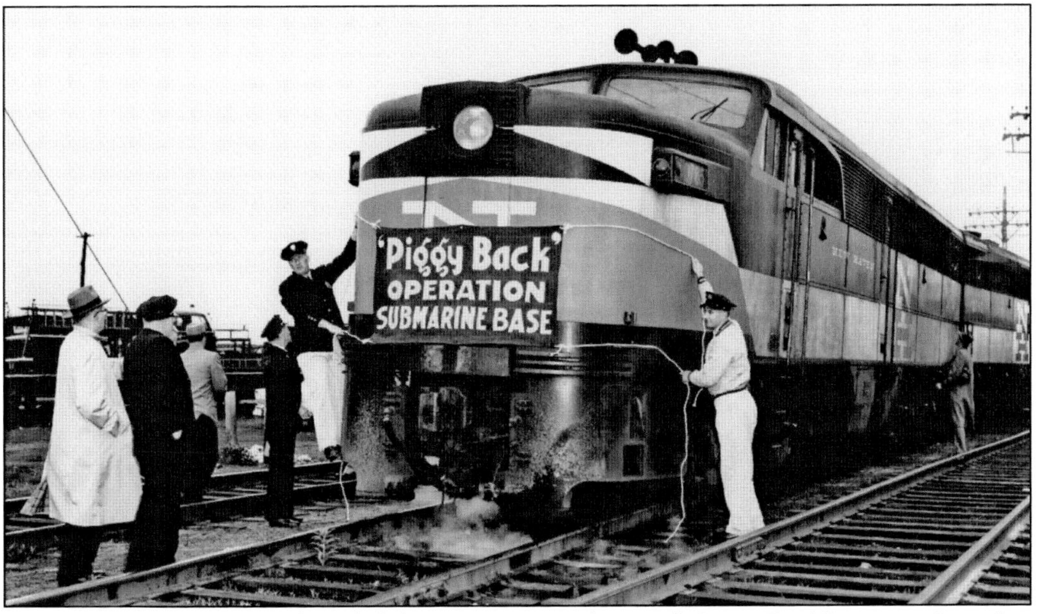

On May 20, 1957, a special civil defense exercise nicknamed "Piggy Back" was conducted at Submarine Base New London in Groton. The purpose of the drill was to test the mobility of emergency forces throughout the state in an emergency situation. Fire departments from throughout Connecticut participated, and through the cooperation of the New Haven Railroad, 15 pieces of fire equipment were transported to the submarine base on special flatcars. The engine of the car that transported the equipment is pictured here. (Submarine Base New London Fire Department.)

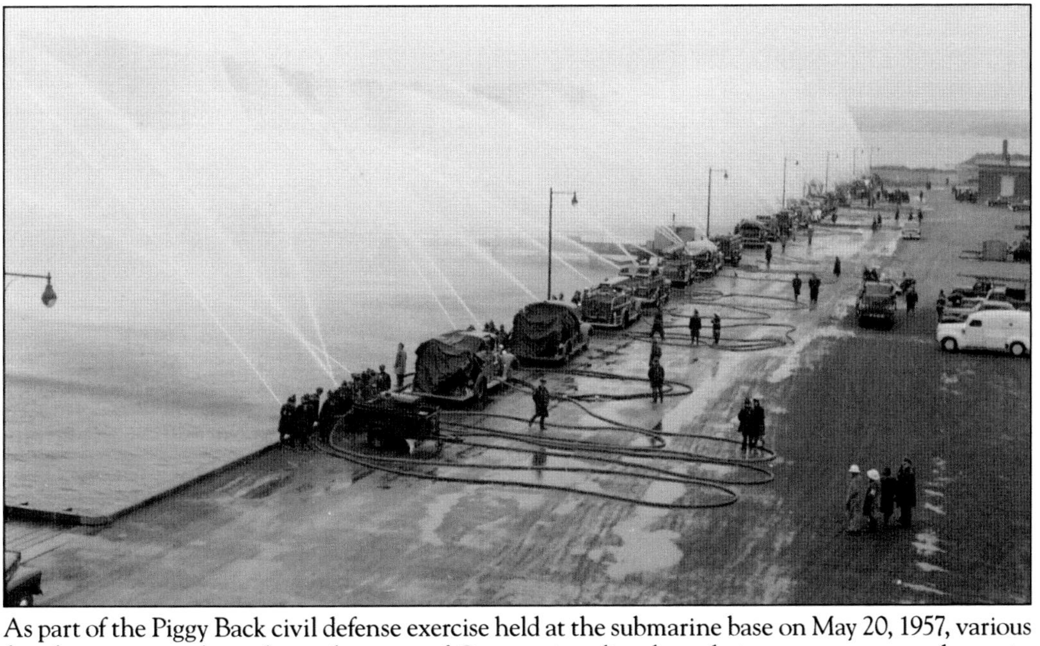

As part of the Piggy Back civil defense exercise held at the submarine base on May 20, 1957, various fire departments throughout the state of Connecticut lined up their apparatuses on the main dock at the base and tested their ability to coordinate firefighting activities during an emergency. Shown in this photograph are various fire department pumper trucks in simultaneous operation to test water flow capabilities at the base. (Rob Palmer.)

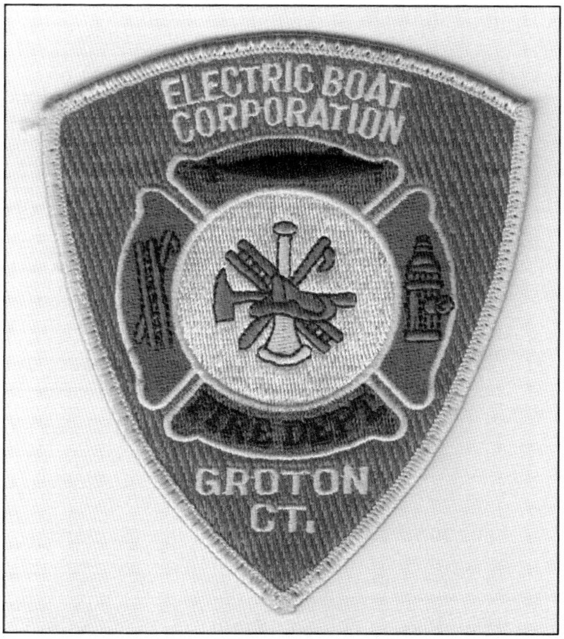

When Electric Boat was established in Groton in 1911, fire protection at the shipyard was provided by a volunteer fire brigade comprised of Electric Boat employees. In the late 1950s, it was determined that a career force was needed, so a staff was hired. Today, the department maintains a modern fire station on Eastern Point Road with a career force capable of performing high-angle rescue, confined-space rescue, and rapid dewatering; handling hazardous materials incidents; and providing firefighting and emergency medical services. (Electric Boat Fire Department.)

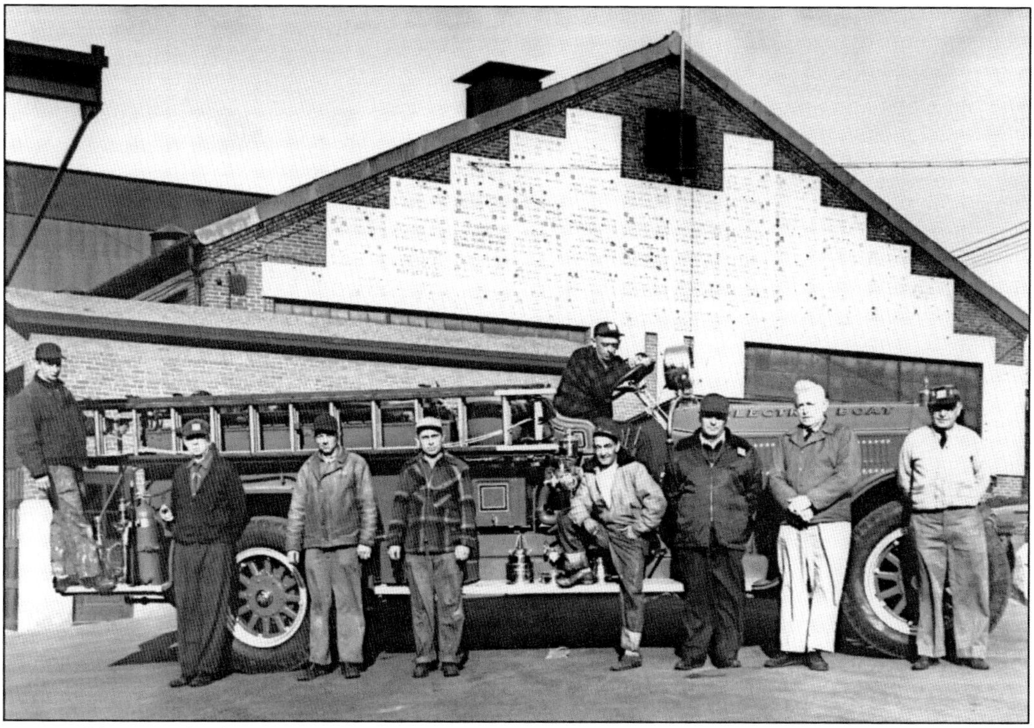

Pictured here with Electric Boat's newly acquired 1929 Ward LaFrance engine in the late 1940s are the first shift men who manned it. From left to right are (standing in front of truck) Thomas Wakely, Harry Muscarella, Ralph Kilpatrick, Joseph Sequara, Albert Musante, Chief Thomas O'Niell, and John Ullrich; (on truck) Stephen Powaleny and Driver Peter Procko. Note the white signs on the building behind the truck; each one represents a submarine built in the shipyard during World War II. (Electric Boat Fire Department.)

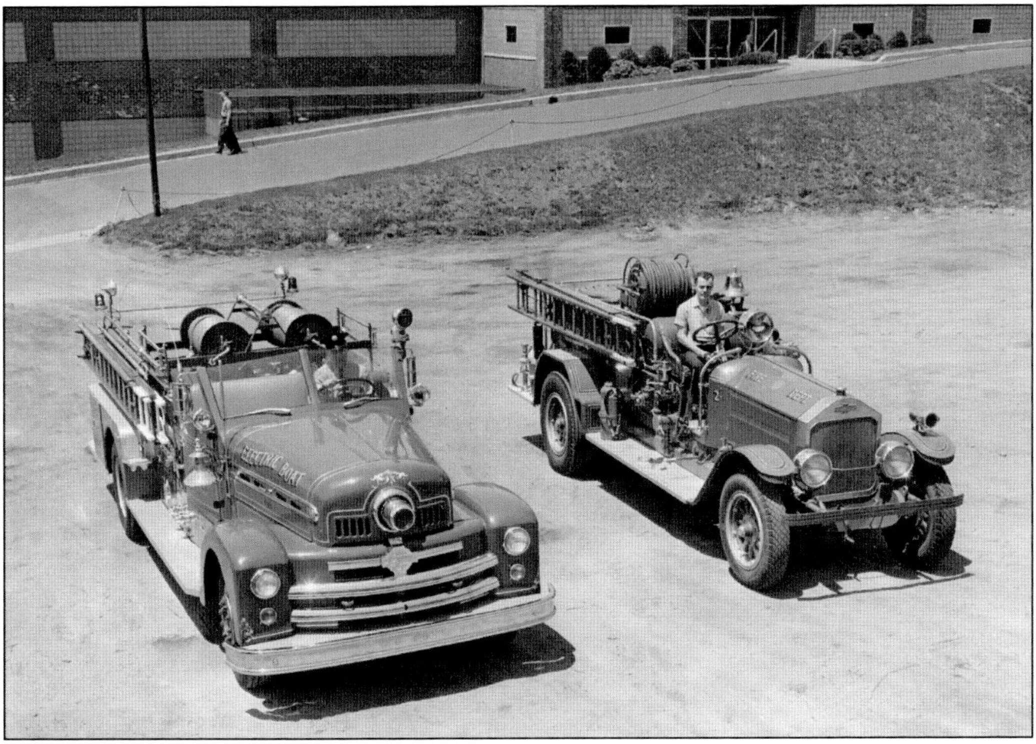

This mid-1950s photograph shows two Electric Boat fire trucks. At left is a 1949 Seagrave engine driven by Robert Sawyer, and at right is a 1929 Ward LaFrance with an unknown volunteer driver. Electric Boat donated the Ward LaFrance to the Eastern Connecticut Fire Training School sometime in the late 1960s or early 1970s. (Electric Boat Fire Department.)

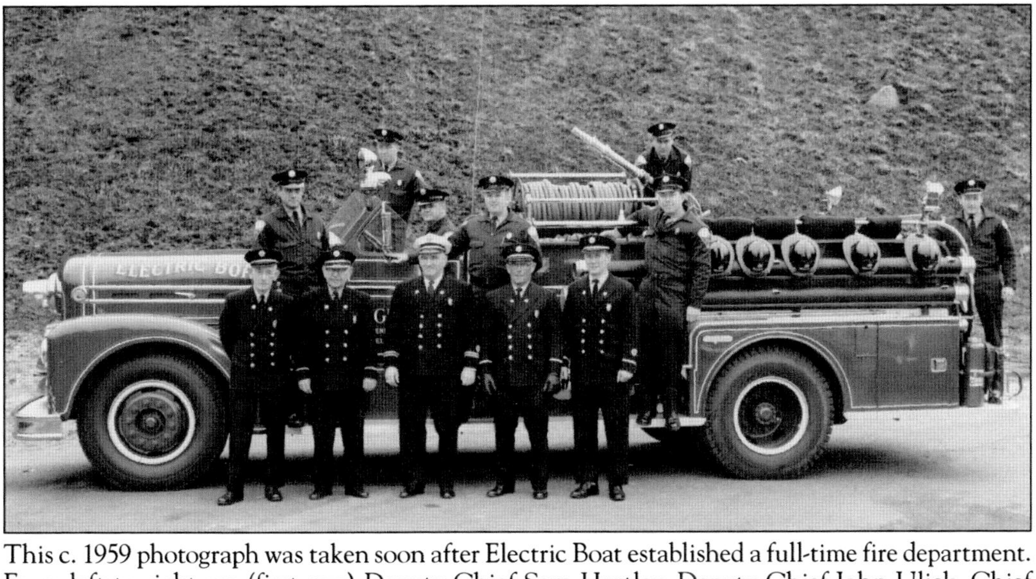

This c. 1959 photograph was taken soon after Electric Boat established a full-time fire department. From left to right are (first row) Deputy Chief Sam Hartley, Deputy Chief John Ulick, Chief Clifford Parks, Deputy Chief Frank Pollard, and Deputy Chief George Fargo; (second row) Doug Black, Robert Hill (driver), William Nott, and Richard Jansen; (on top of truck) Felix Brochu and Robert Sawyer; (on back of truck) James Arnold. (Electric Boat Fire Department.)

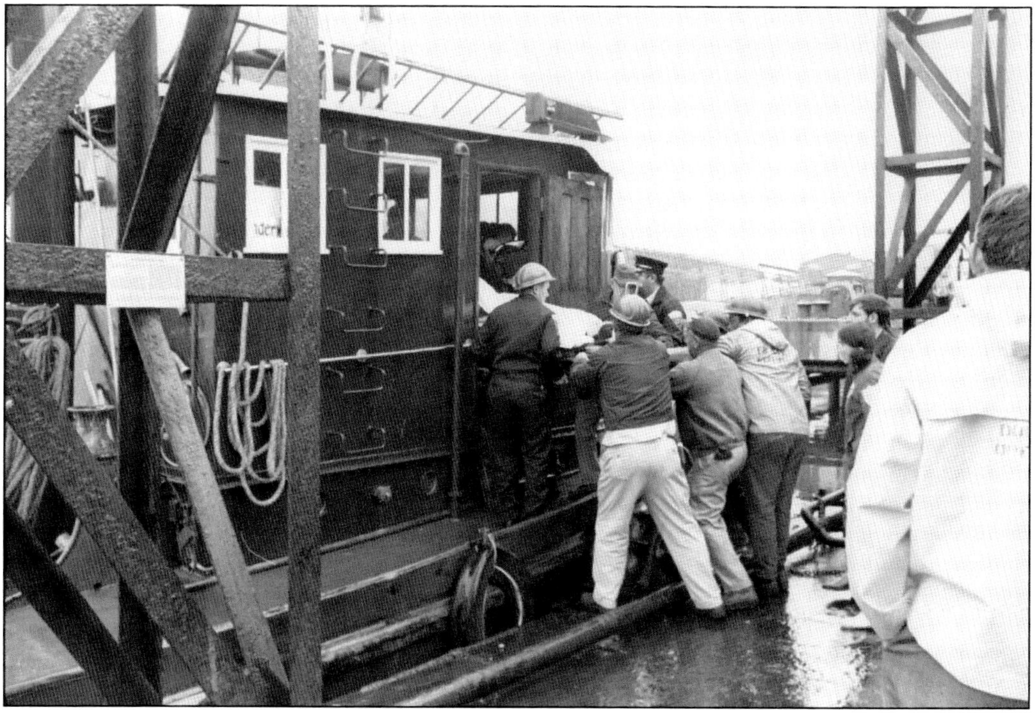

In the 1960s, when only one Gold Star Bridge existed, contingencies were made to transport patients from Electric Boat to Lawrence + Memorial Hospital in New London. In the event that the bridge was shut down, tugboats were utilized. After the boat had crossed the river, a New London ambulance would finish transporting patients to the hospital. This photograph was taken sometime around 1969. (Electric Boat Fire Department.)

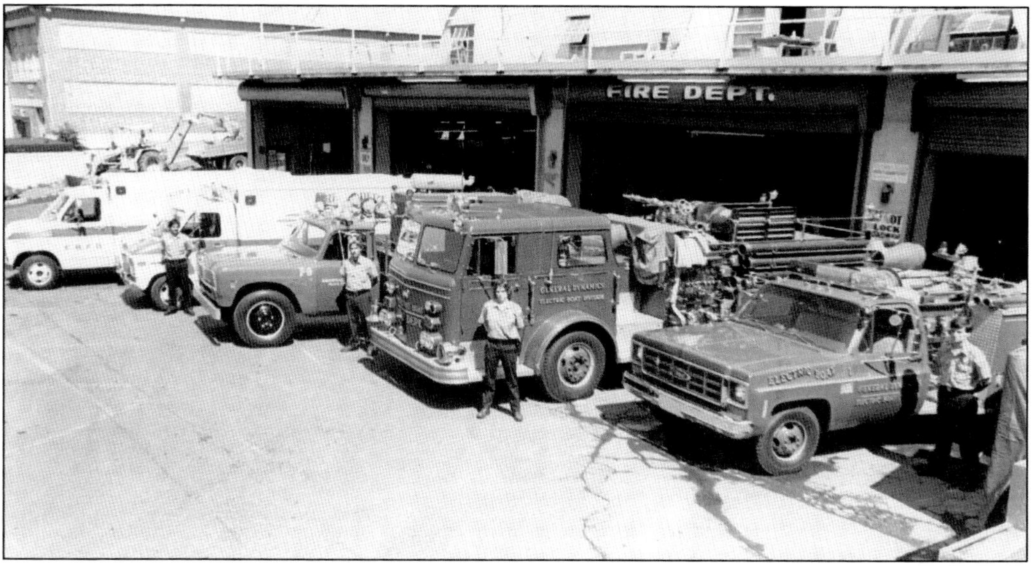

Parked in front of the old fire station located inside the yard is Electric Boat's 1980s fleet, which included two ambulances, a dewatering truck, a Class A engine, and a mini pumper. From left to right are Mark Springer, Mark Melanson, Bridget Yuknat, and Charles Chaffee. (Electric Boat Fire Department.)

The Charles Pfizer Company purchased Groton's Victory Shipyard in 1947. The current Pfizer firehouse began as the Victory Yard station in 1947. The fire brigade, which started in 1948, peaked at about 70 personnel, and the career department organized in 1949. Today, the department keeps its equipment and skills current and provides dedicated service to both Pfizer and the surrounding community. (Pfizer Fire Department.)

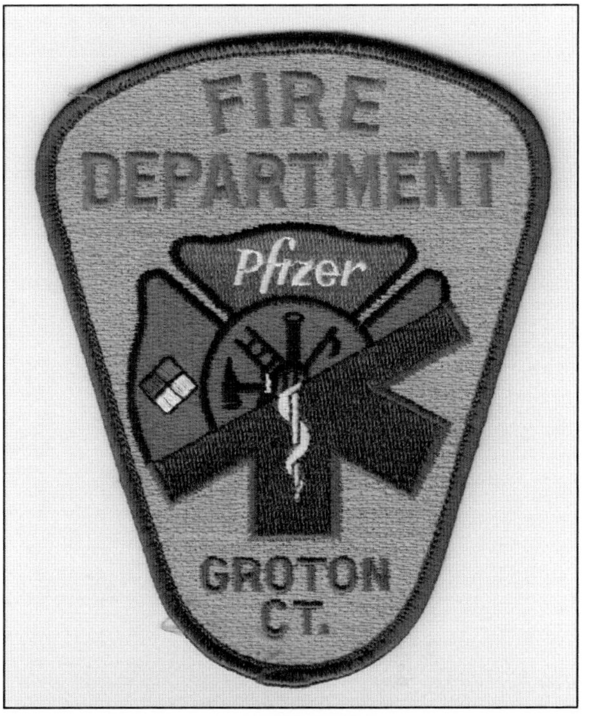

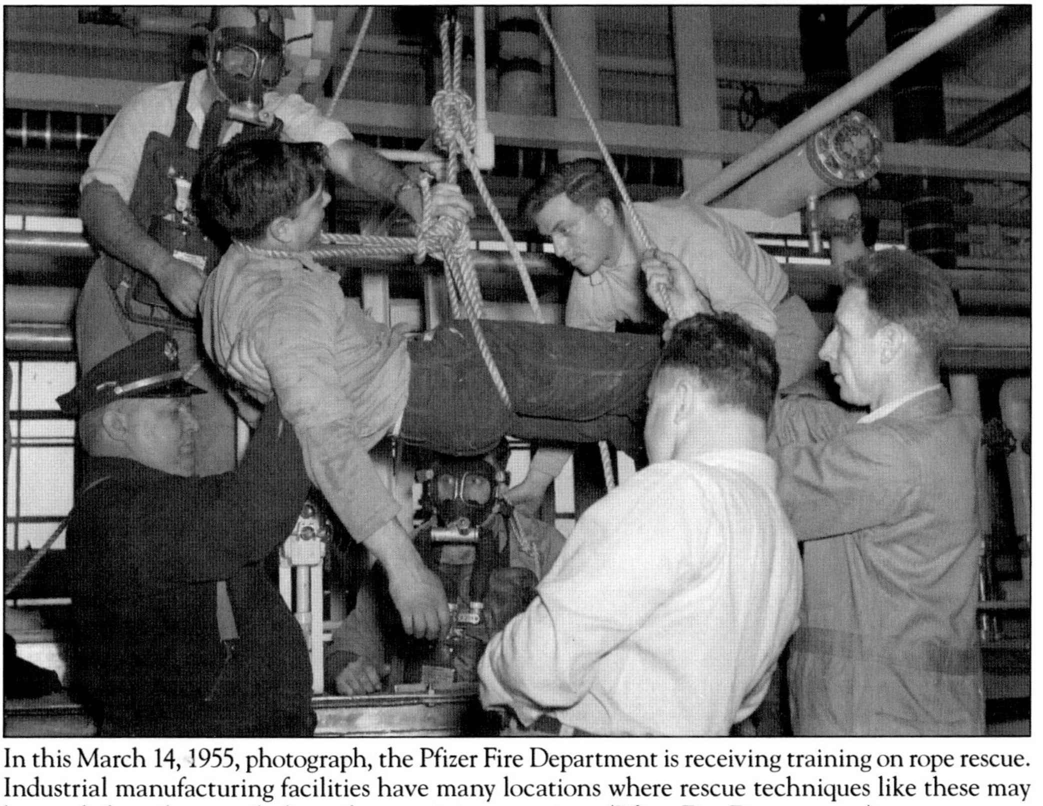

In this March 14, 1955, photograph, the Pfizer Fire Department is receiving training on rope rescue. Industrial manufacturing facilities have many locations where rescue techniques like these may be needed, so they regularly perform training exercises. (Pfizer Fire Department.)

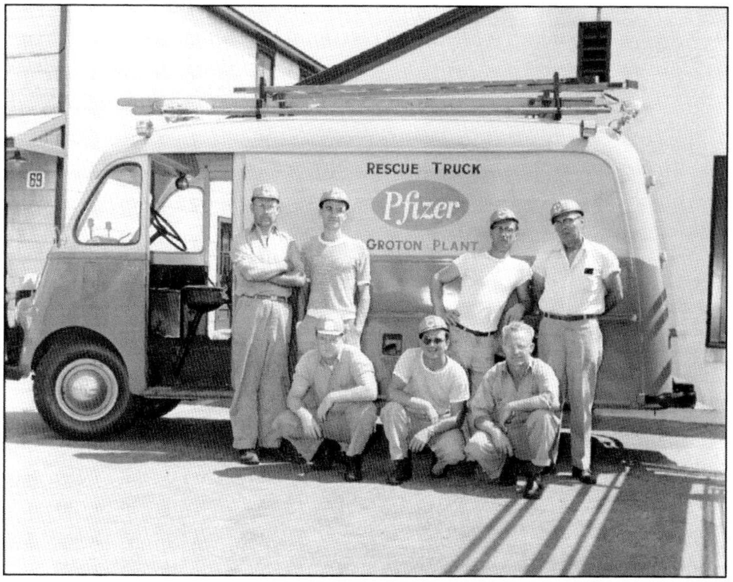

Members of the Pfizer Fire Department stand with their new rescue van in July 1956. Specialized equipment of that time was carried on-board. The concept proved its worth, as the van was replaced in 1970 and has been updated several times since then. (Pfizer Fire Department.)

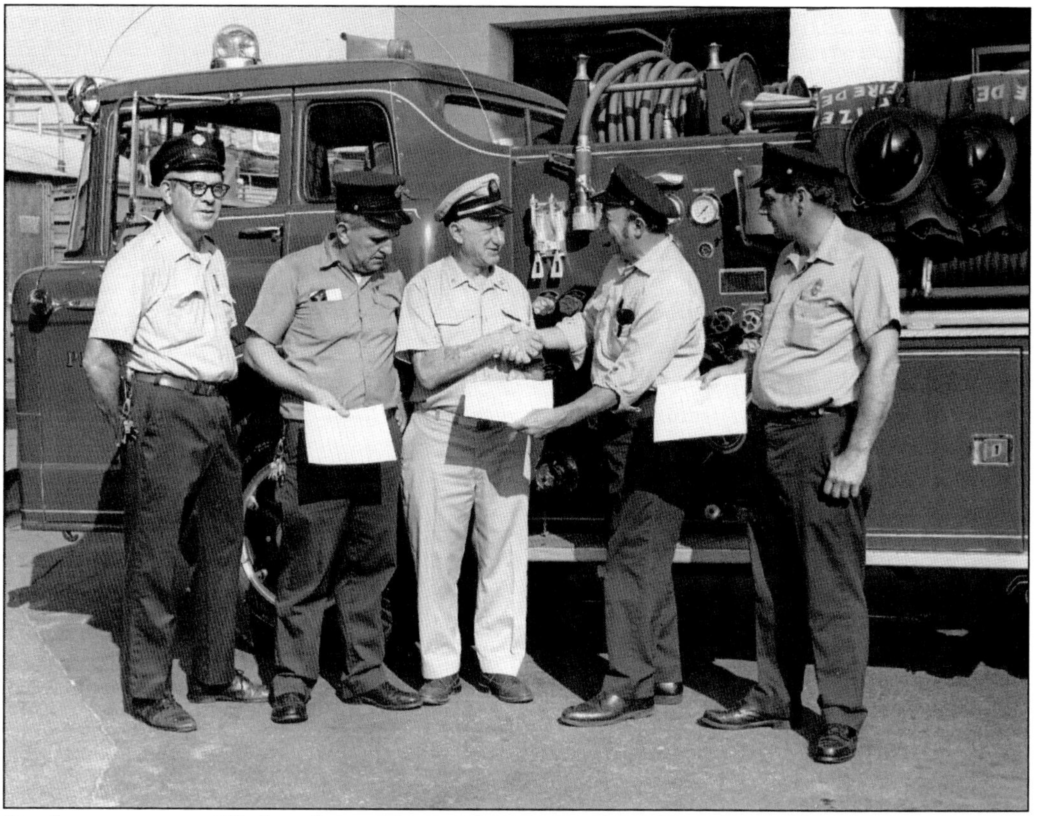

On four successive Wednesdays in September 1975, Pfizer firefighters trained at the Eastern Connecticut Fire Training School in Willimantic. From left to right are Fire Marshal Earl Burke, Robert Johns, instructor Chief Leno Vescovi, Al Duplice, and Ray Christian. According to Chief Vescovi, "It is a great relief to know that this group, rarely noticed but always there, are constantly updating their knowledge of firefighting techniques." (Pfizer Fire Department.)

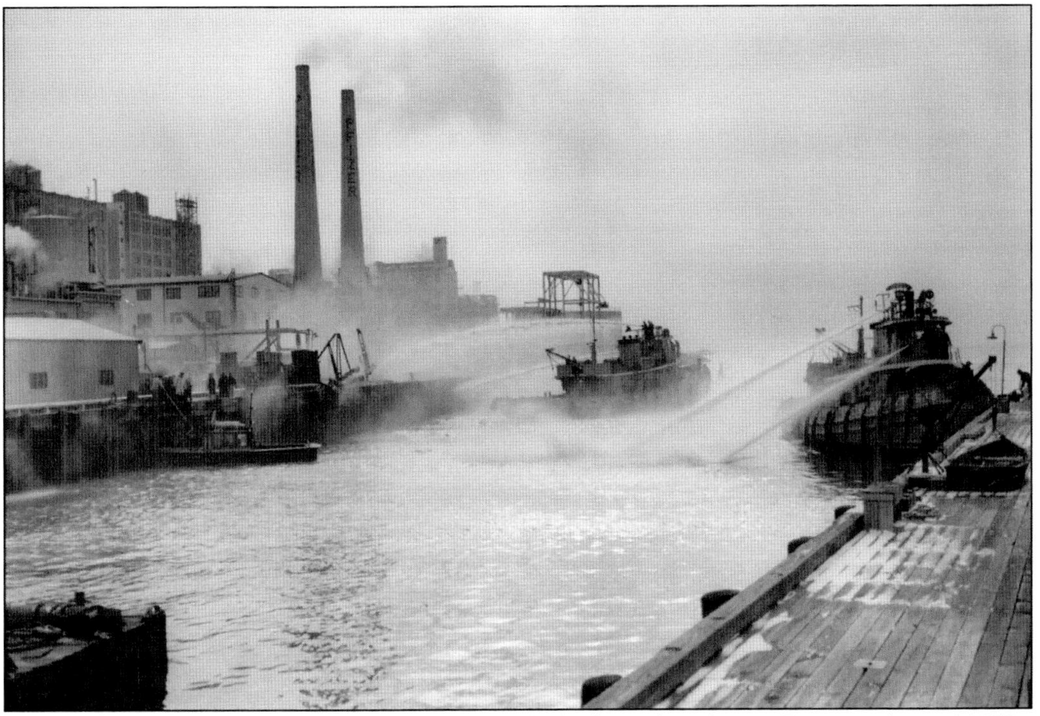

Pfizer firefighters battle a fire on the company's dock along the Thames River in the mid-1950s. Civilian and US Navy tugboats use master streams to help extinguish the fire and dilute any possible chemicals that might have entered the river. (Pfizer Fire Department.)

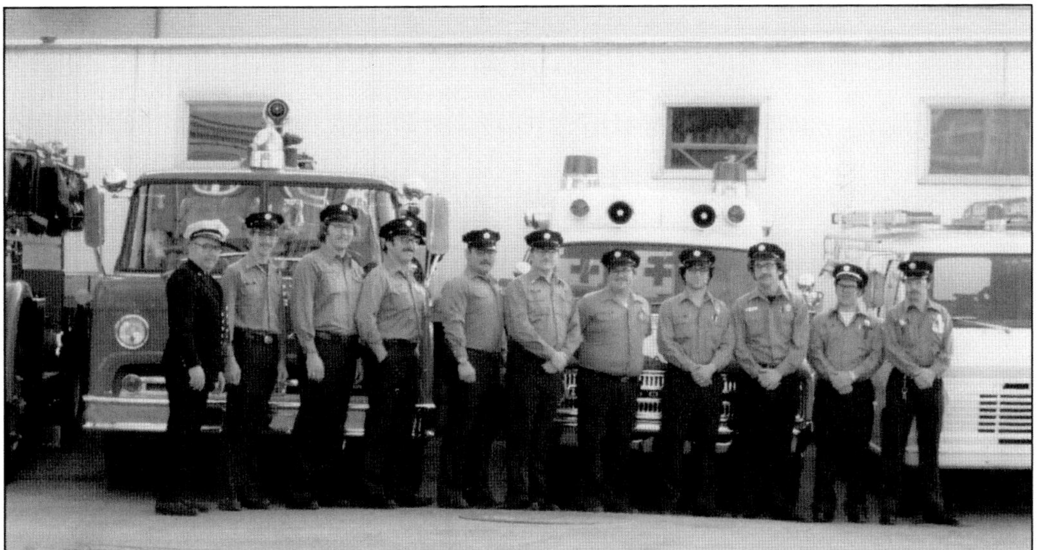

Pfizer Fire Department personnel pose with their fleet in September 1981. From left to right are Chief Ray Schaffer, Jim Fonner, Chris McCormack, William Toby, Greg Mankiewicz, Spike Perkins, Gary Pinkham, Joe Froio, Mark Senior, Art Wheeler, and Ed Brailey. The engine on the far left, a 1979 International/National Foam Company vehicle, was the first unit they purchased to department specifications. It replaced a 1942 Chevrolet carbon-dioxide truck that was left to them when they took possession of the Victory Shipyard. (Pfizer Fire Department.)

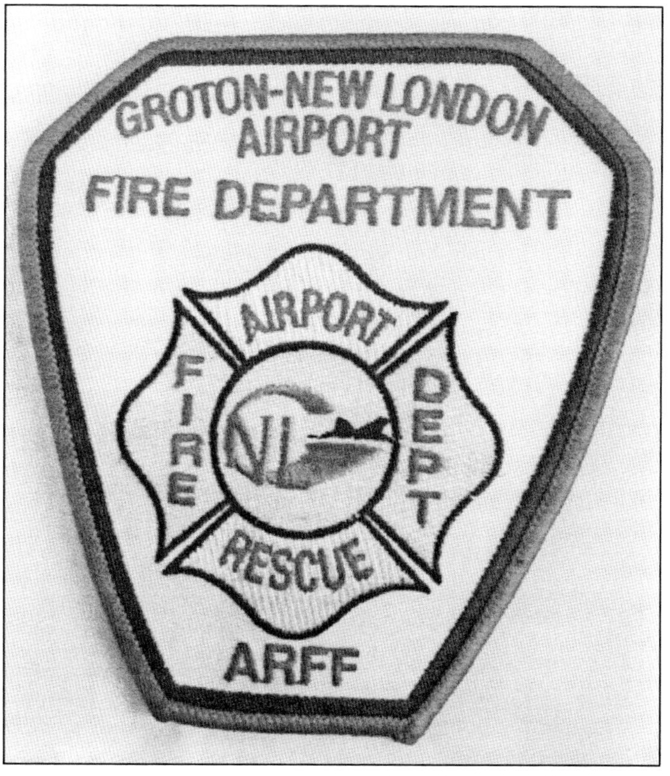

The Groton–New London Airport is a small, publicly owned facility that provides services to corporate and other privately owned aircraft, as well as support for the Army National Guard's 1109th TASMG (Theater Aviation Sustainment Maintenance Group) military aircraft. The airport's fire department is equipped with apparatuses provided by the State of Connecticut. Personnel assigned to the fire department are also assigned to security and facility maintenance tasks at the airport; the department provides an initial response to fires and other emergencies on the 489-acre site until the arrival of equipment and personnel from various Groton and Mystic fire departments. (Groton–New London Airport.)

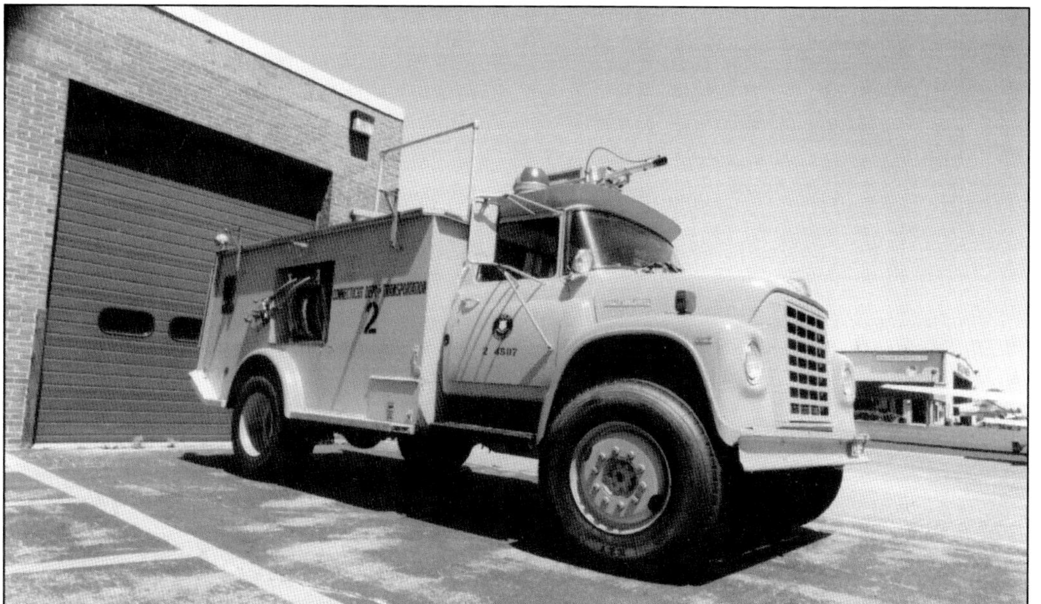

This International crash truck, which carries 1,350 pounds of dry chemical powder and 250 gallons of premixed foam and water, has served the airport since the mid-1960s. The truck, pictured here around 1970, is a six-wheel drive and has the ability to flow foam through the turret on the roof of the cab. (Groton–New London Airport.)

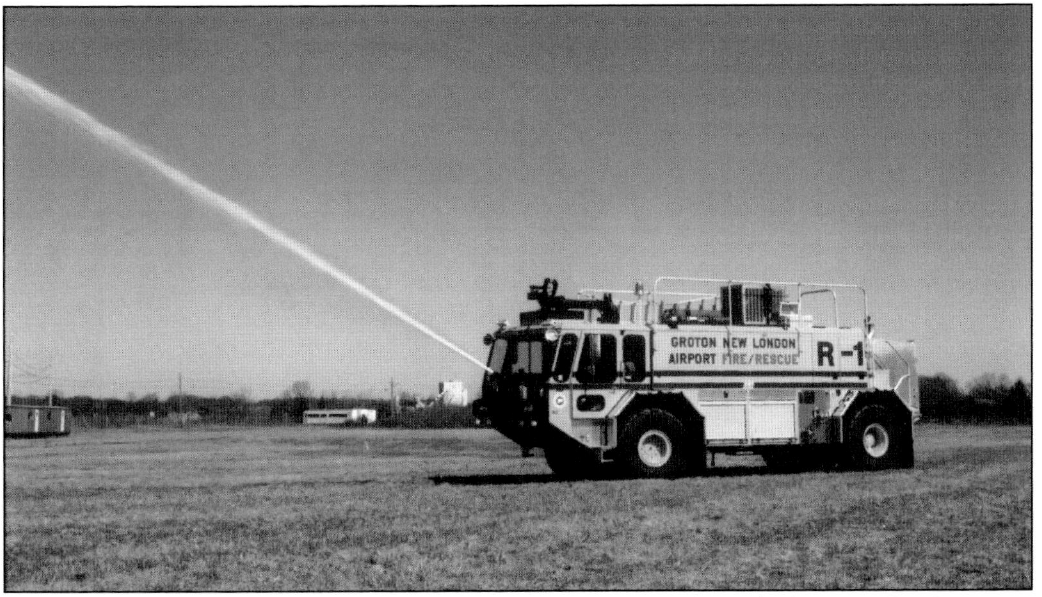

Shown in this c. 2000 photograph is a 1998 E-One Titan crash truck designated as Rescue-1. The truck carries 1,500 gallons of water, 200 gallons of foam, and 500 pounds of dry chemicals. It was removed from service in 2012. (Groton–New London Airport.)

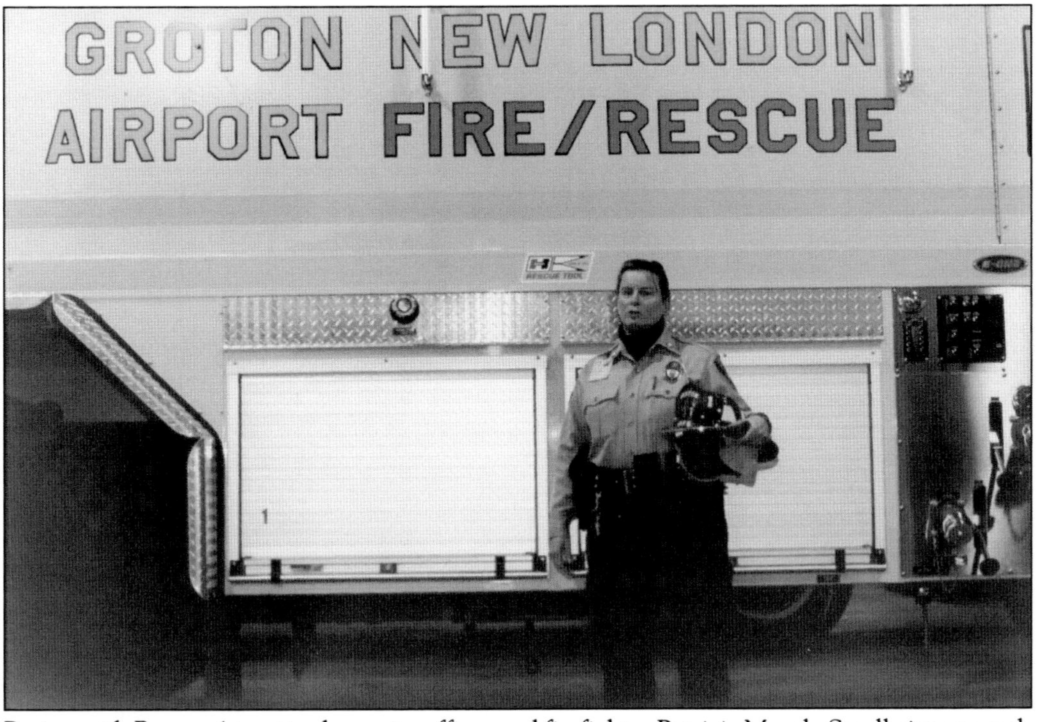

Posing with Rescue-1 is retired security officer and firefighter Patricia Macek. Small airports such as Groton–New London do not have personnel strictly assigned to firefighting; the staff is also tasked with providing support to the security or maintenance departments within the airport. Any structural fires on the property would be handled by the civilian fire departments in town. (Groton–New London Airport.)

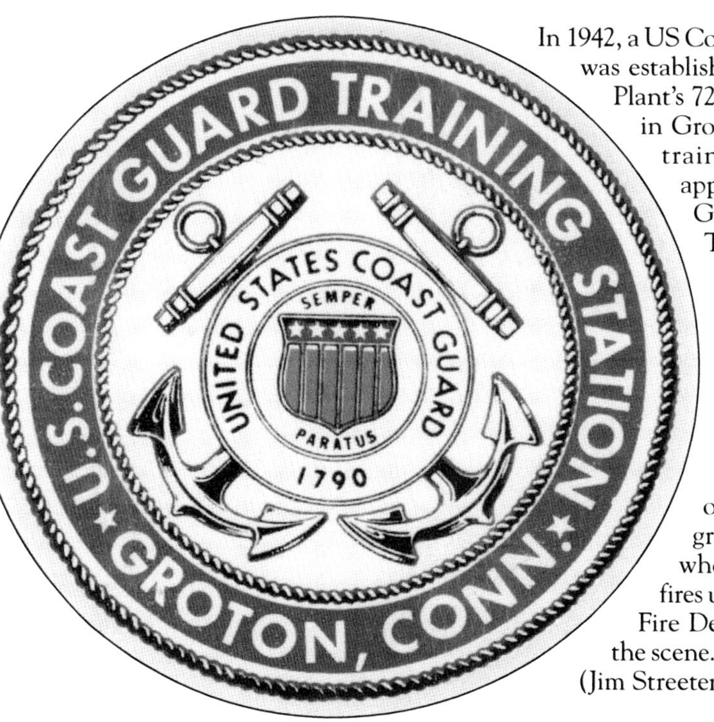

In 1942, a US Coast Guard Training Station was established on the former Morton Plant's 72-acre estate at Avery Point in Groton. The station provided training in various skills to approximately 20,000 Coast Guard personnel each year. There were approximately 40 buildings on the property, many of which were constructed of wood. Because of the number of buildings and personnel assigned to the station, a small fire department was necessary. It was comprised of one fire truck and a small group of Coast Guard men who would respond to small fires until the Borough of Groton Fire Department could arrive on the scene. The station closed in 1967. (Jim Streeter.)

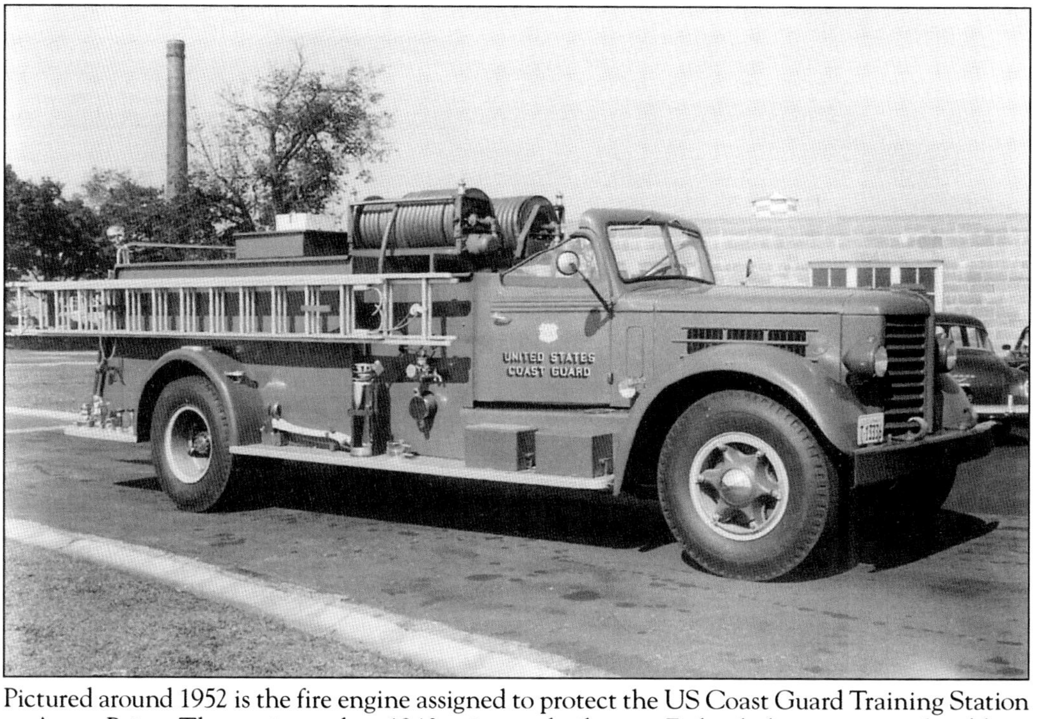

Pictured around 1952 is the fire engine assigned to protect the US Coast Guard Training Station at Avery Point. The engine, a late-1940s vintage built on a Federal chassis, was utilized by a brigade made up of Coast Guard personnel. Vehicles like this were purchased in bulk from various manufacturers by the federal government during World War II. Many of them were later used in civilian service after they were sold as surplus. (Jim Streeter.)

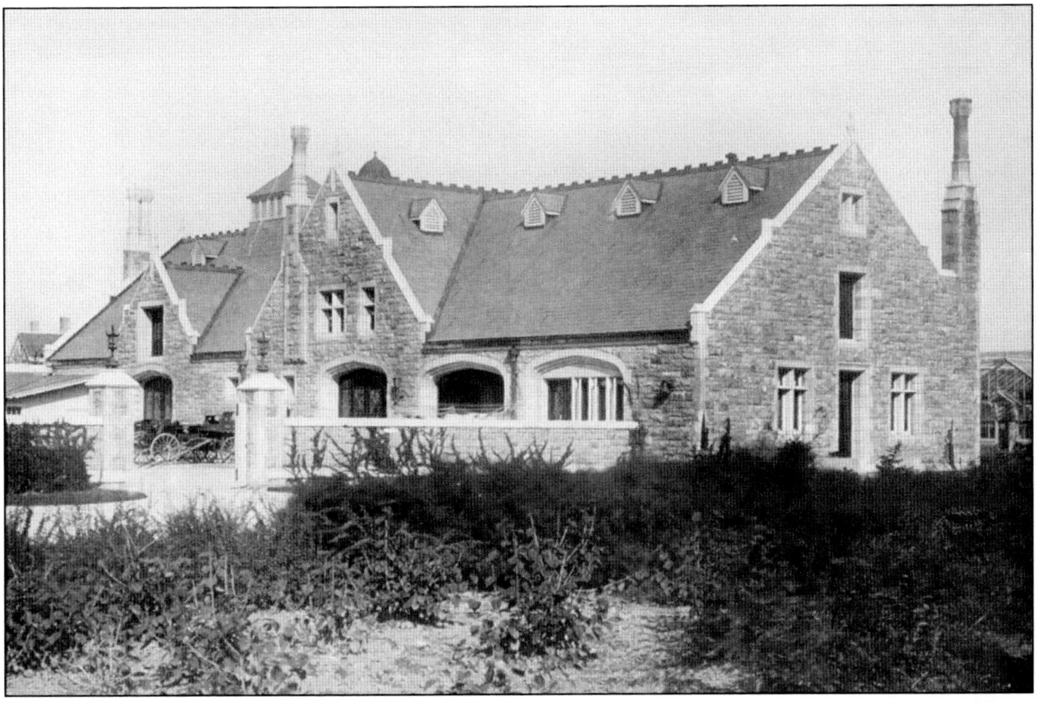

The US Coast Guard used the granite barn and garage at the former Plant Estate (pictured here around 1903) as their fire station. Personnel assigned as firefighters used the second story of this building as sleeping quarters. Today, it is used as a maintenance facility for the University of Connecticut at Avery Point. (Jim Streeter.)

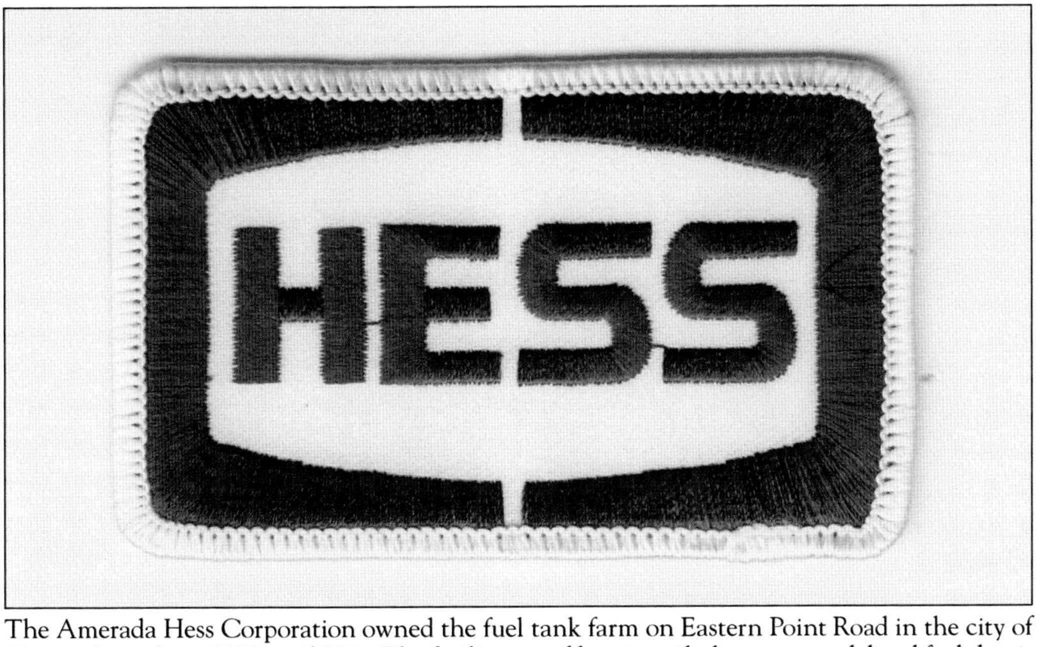

The Amerada Hess Corporation owned the fuel tank farm on Eastern Point Road in the city of Groton from about 1970 until 2014. The facility stored heating oils, kerosene, and diesel fuel that it received by barge on the Thames River. Deeming it necessary to have fire protection, Hess assigned a firefighting vehicle to the terminal and trained the staff in fire protection. (William Tischer.)

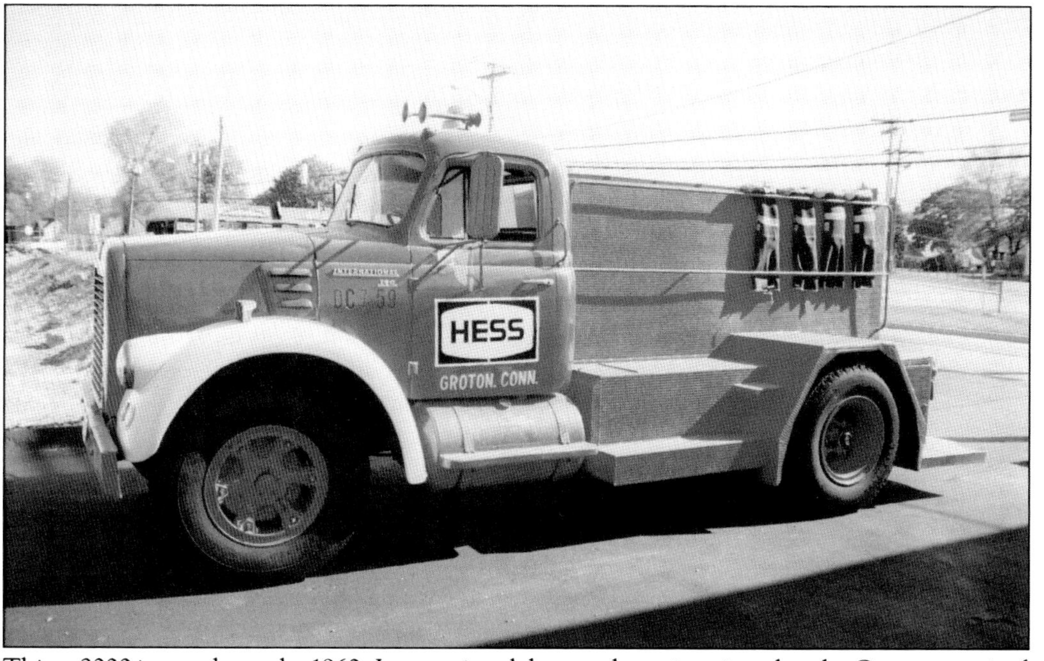

This c. 2000 image shows the 1960s International dry powder unit assigned to the Groton terminal owned by Hess Corporation. It carried several dry powder cylinders that were propelled by carbon dioxide. The vehicle was used by trained employees as a first response to an emergency until the City of Groton Fire Department could arrive. (William Tischer.)

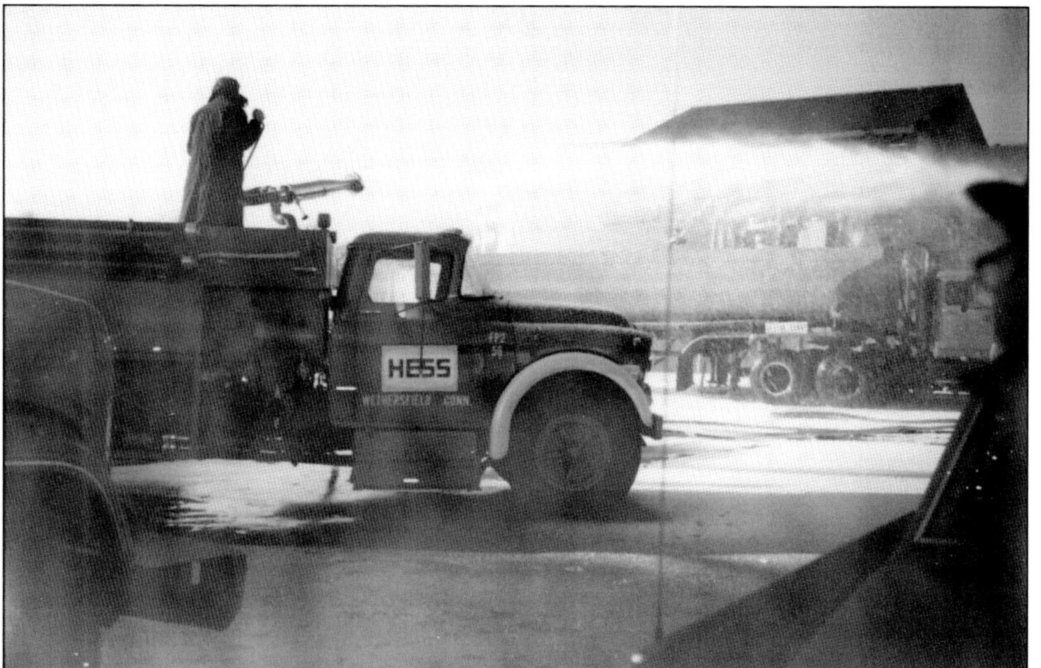

Here, Hess employees are being trained in how to fight fuel oil fires. The training was conducted at a Hess facility in Wethersfield, Connecticut. (Gary Rassmussen and Mike Malley.)

Three

Police Departments

The City of Groton and the Groton Long Point fire districts have their own forms of governing bodies. Although residents of both districts pay property taxes to the Town of Groton and as such are entitled to services provided by the Town of Groton Police Department, each has elected to have, and pay for, their own dedicated, organized police department to serve the residents within their districts.

It should be noted that historically, the Town of Groton has contributed a large portion of the cost of the annual police budgets in the City of Groton and Groton Long Point.

According to a report from a November 2013 police study, the Town of Groton Police Department is staffed with a total of 67 sworn officers and has jurisdiction throughout the entire town, including the two districts that provide their own separate police services. The City of Groton's department has a staff of 29 sworn officers, and Groton Long Point, which has a residential population that increases dramatically in the summer months, is staffed with five full-time and four part-time sworn officers. Both the City of Groton and Groton Long Point officers have police powers only within the jurisdiction of their districts. All the police officers representing these departments are well trained and perform professionally at their assigned tasks.

The issue of consolidating the three police departments has been a topic of discussion over the last 50-plus years, and many studies have been conducted to determine the pros and cons of doing so. Although some studies indicate that it is possible that tax savings could be realized by consolidating the departments, much resistance has been voiced from residents in both the City of Groton and Groton Long Point who enjoy the "extra" and dedicated services they receive from their own police departments.

From 1923 until 1973, the Connecticut State Police maintained one of the state's seven police stations/barracks here in Groton. State troopers have jurisdiction throughout the state, including Groton, and have provided assistance to the police in the Town of Groton throughout the years.

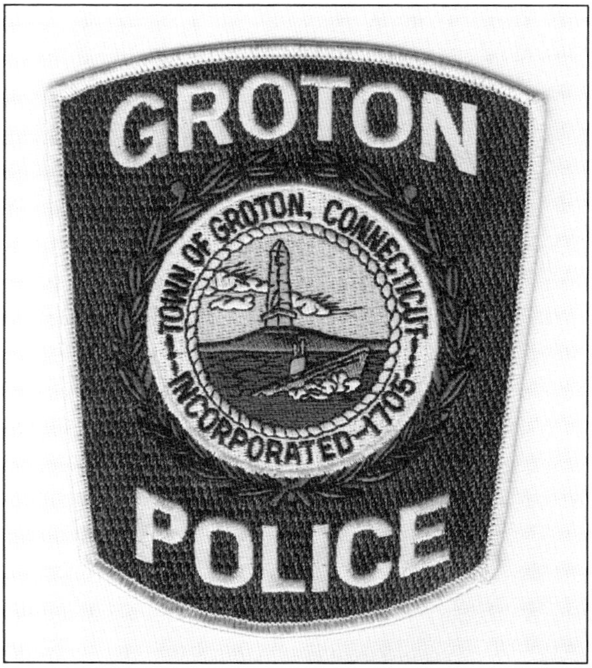

The Town of Groton Police Department can trace it roots back to 1900, when three men were appointed by the town and given the title of patrolmen. These patrolmen did not receive a set salary and only worked when called upon. In 1935, the town hired its first regularly paid patrolmen. In 1939, the Connecticut Legislature passed an act that officially approved an organized police department in the town; at the time, there were three regularly paid officers. Over the years, the Town of Groton Police Department has grown considerably, and as of July 2015, the department has a total of 67 sworn officers, including the chief. (Town of Groton Police Department.)

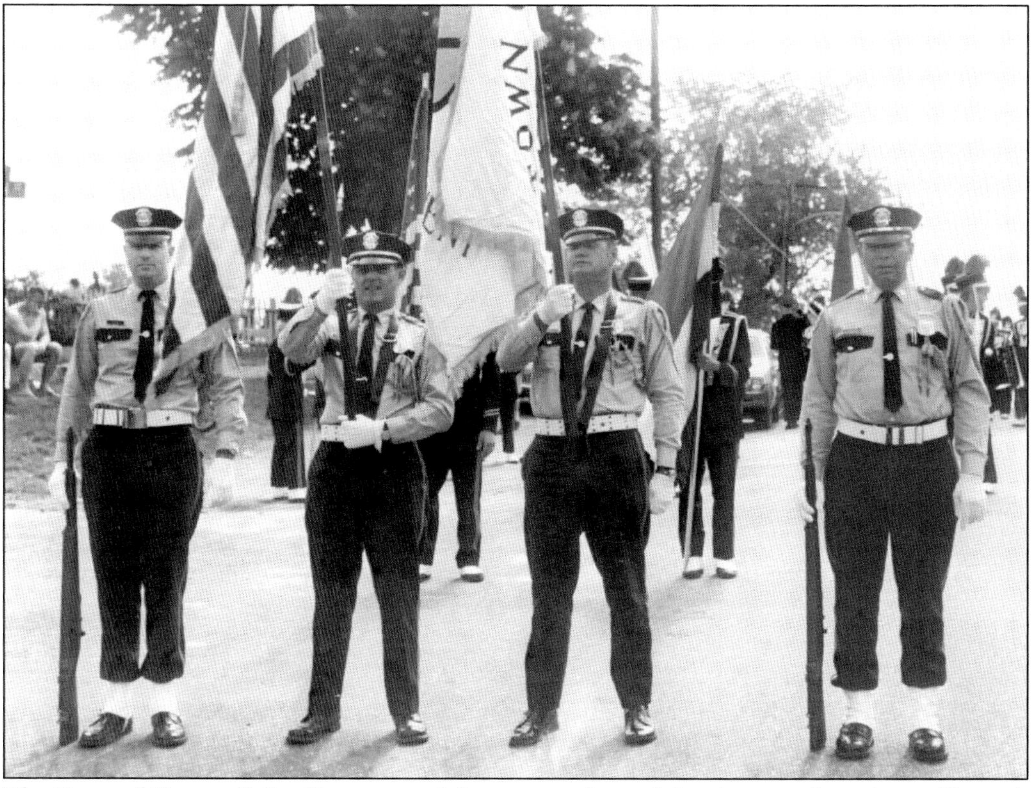

The Town of Groton Police Department's honor guard posed for photographs prior to Groton's 1968 Fourth of July Parade. From left to right are Worley Smith, Vern Crooker, Spencer Havey, and Lawrence Pinette. (Town of Groton Police Department.)

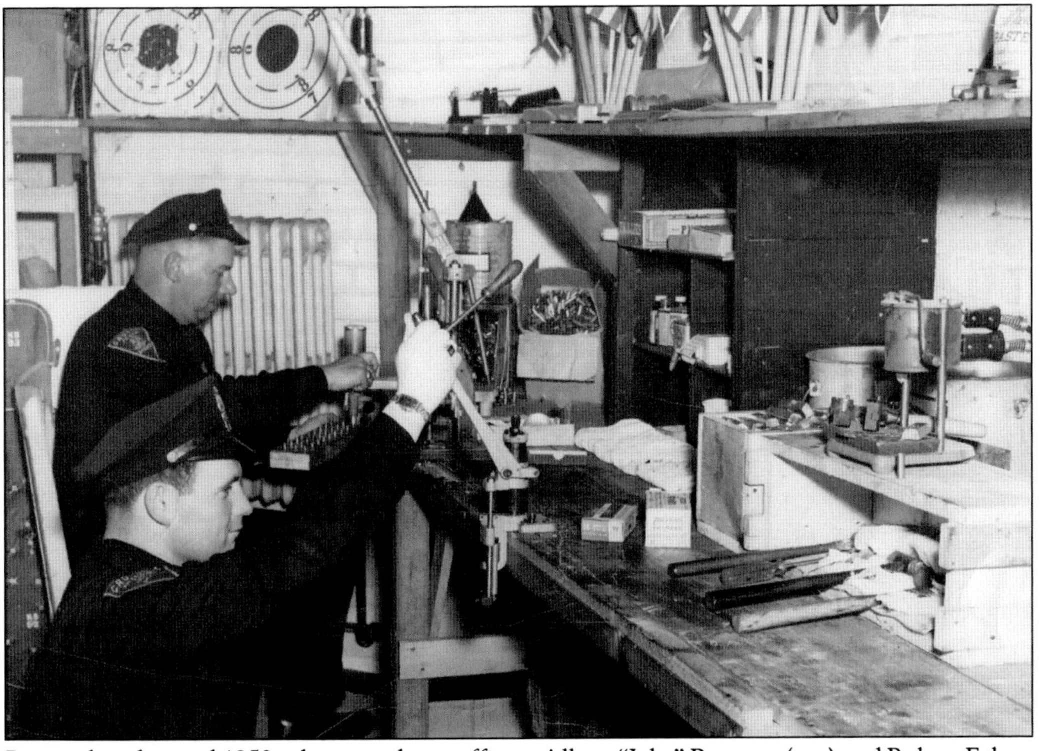

Pictured in this mid-1950s photograph are officers Albert "Jake" Burrows (top) and Robert Falvey reloading ammunition in the police facilities in the basement of the town hall building on Fort Hill Road. The ammunition was used for target practice and to supply members of the department's pistol team. (Town of Groton Police Department.)

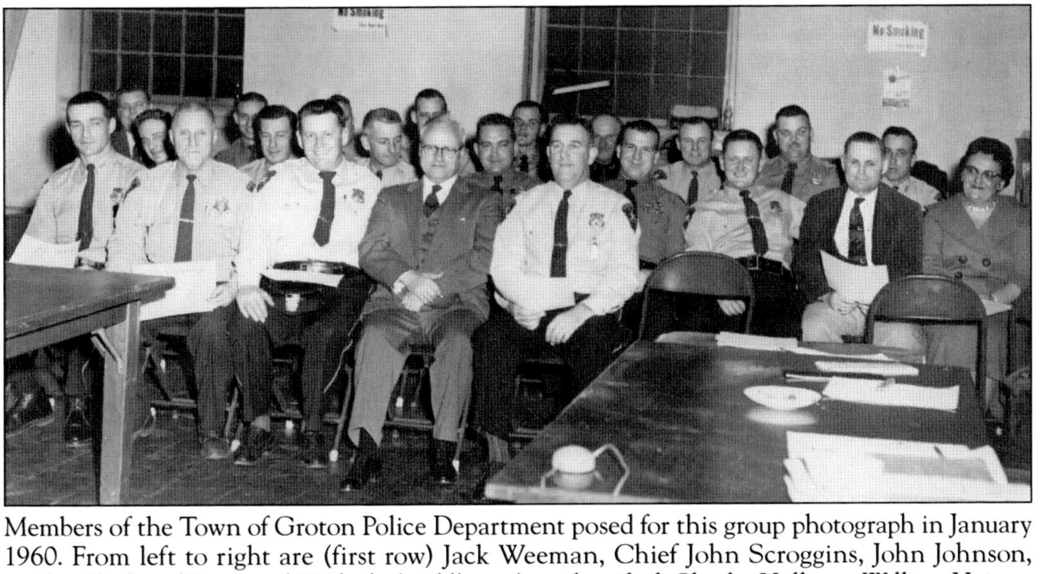

Members of the Town of Groton Police Department posed for this group photograph in January 1960. From left to right are (first row) Jack Weeman, Chief John Scroggins, John Johnson, unidentified, and Raymond Garlock; (middle row) unidentified, Charles Halligan, William Haines, unidentified, Gerald Griffin, Earl Cate, Robert Falvey, and Grace Bjork; (third row) unidentified, Robert Ravenelle, Anthony D'Arcangelo, Orren Merry, Russel Barber, Elbert Palmer, David Falvey, Walter Swan, and Leland Gray. (Beverly Gray.)

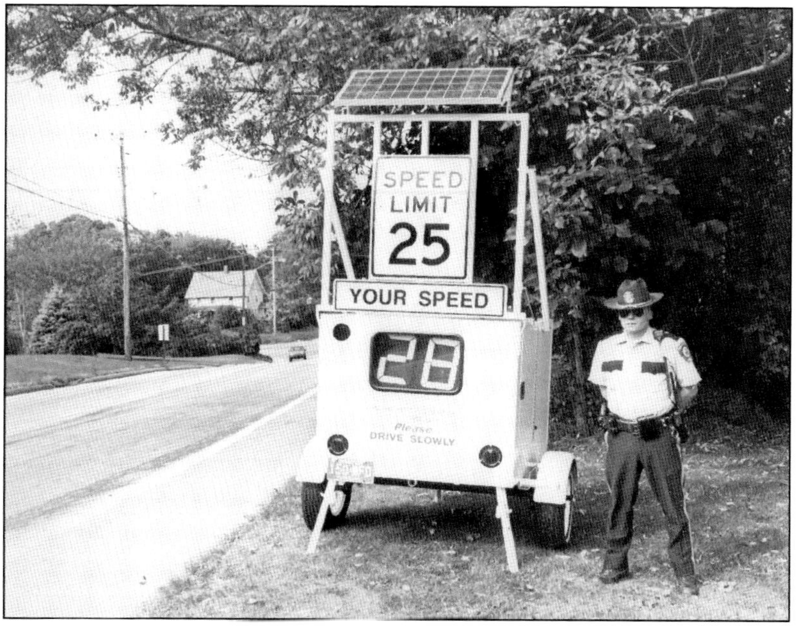

Officer Jay Graves is pictured in this c. 1990 photograph standing next to the department's radar speed sign. The department displays this device on various streets throughout town for traffic control and to promote speed awareness, especially in areas where a number of complaints have been made about speeding vehicles. (Jay Graves.)

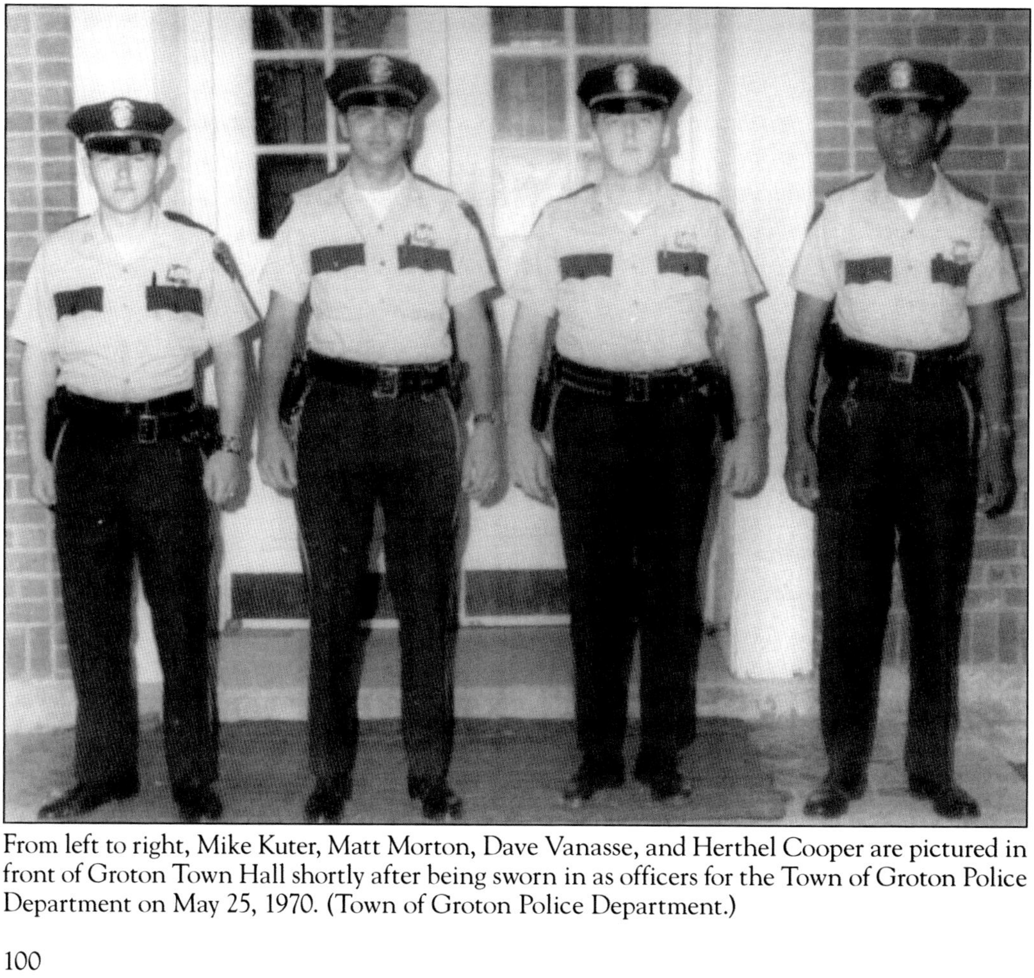

From left to right, Mike Kuter, Matt Morton, Dave Vanasse, and Herthel Cooper are pictured in front of Groton Town Hall shortly after being sworn in as officers for the Town of Groton Police Department on May 25, 1970. (Town of Groton Police Department.)

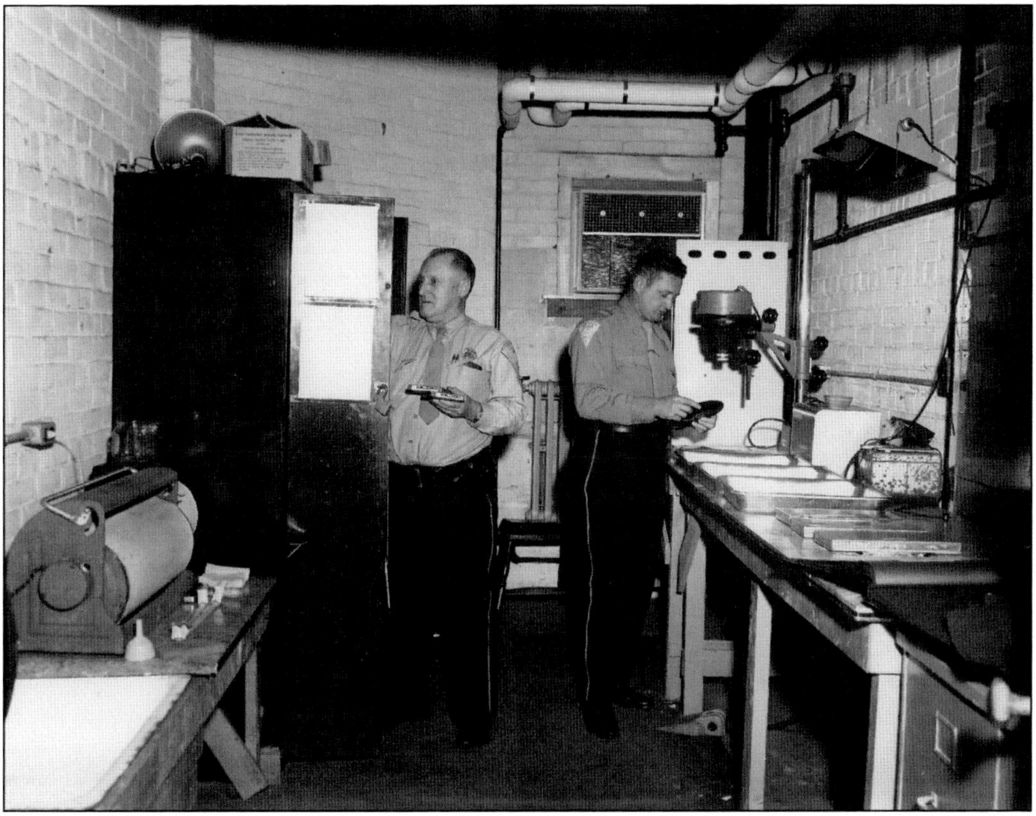

Chief John Scroggins (left) and officer Earl Cate are shown working in the Town of Groton Police Department's photograph-processing laboratory in the late 1950s. Many local departments maintained their own labs as a means of cost savings instead of having the photographs developed and printed commercially. (Town of Groton Police Department.)

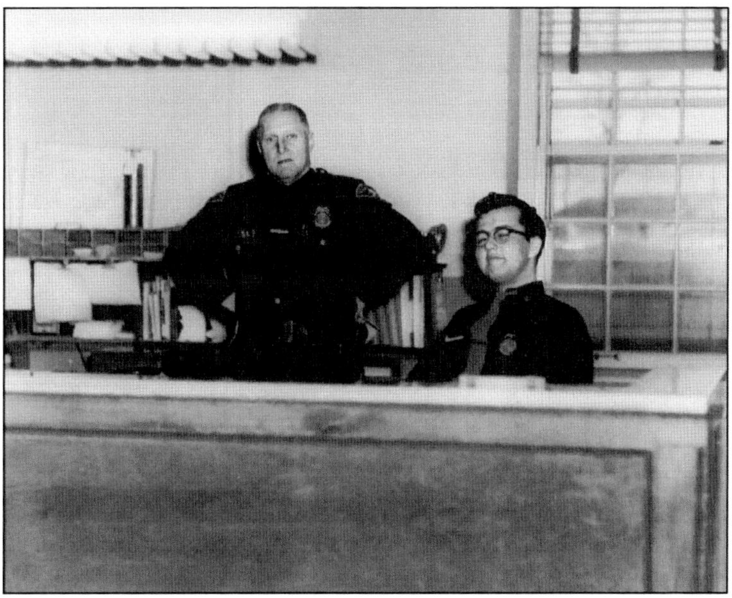

Chief John Scroggins (left) is pictured with Robert Garcia, who was a student at Fitch Senior High School at the time this photograph was taken in 1959. Garcia's class members had voted to have him serve as honorary chief of police for the day at the Town of Groton Police Department. Beginning in 1963, after graduating from high school, Garcia served as a police officer for the Town of Groton Police Department for 15 years. (Town of Groton Police Department.)

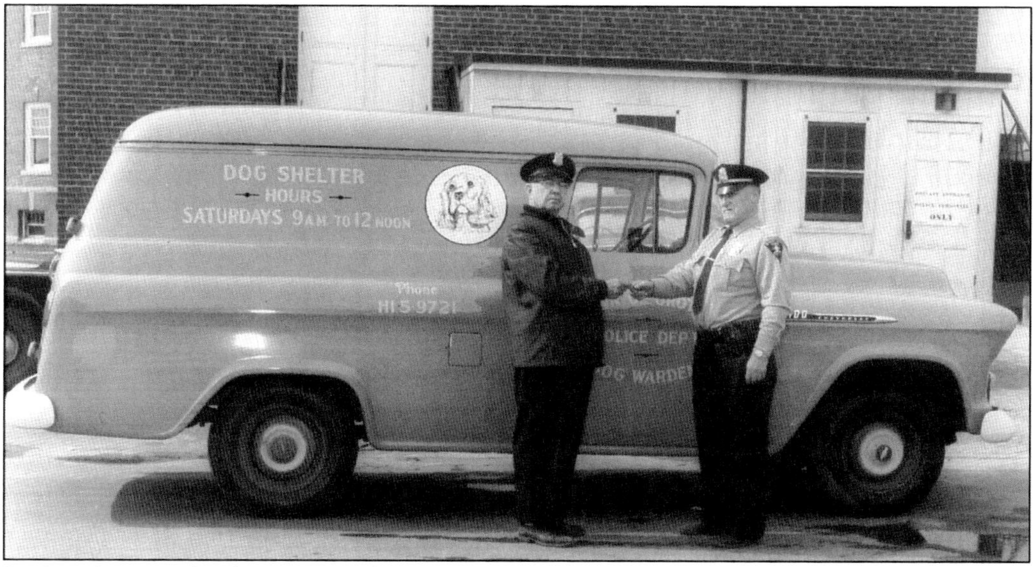
DOG SHELTER
HOURS
SATURDAYS 9AM TO 12 NOON
Phone
HI 5-9721

In this photograph taken on March 30, 1960, Chief John Scroggins (right) is handing the keys to the department's newly acquired 1956 panel truck to dog warden Frank Phillips. Phillips used the vehicle as the town's animal control vehicle. (Town of Groton Police Department.)

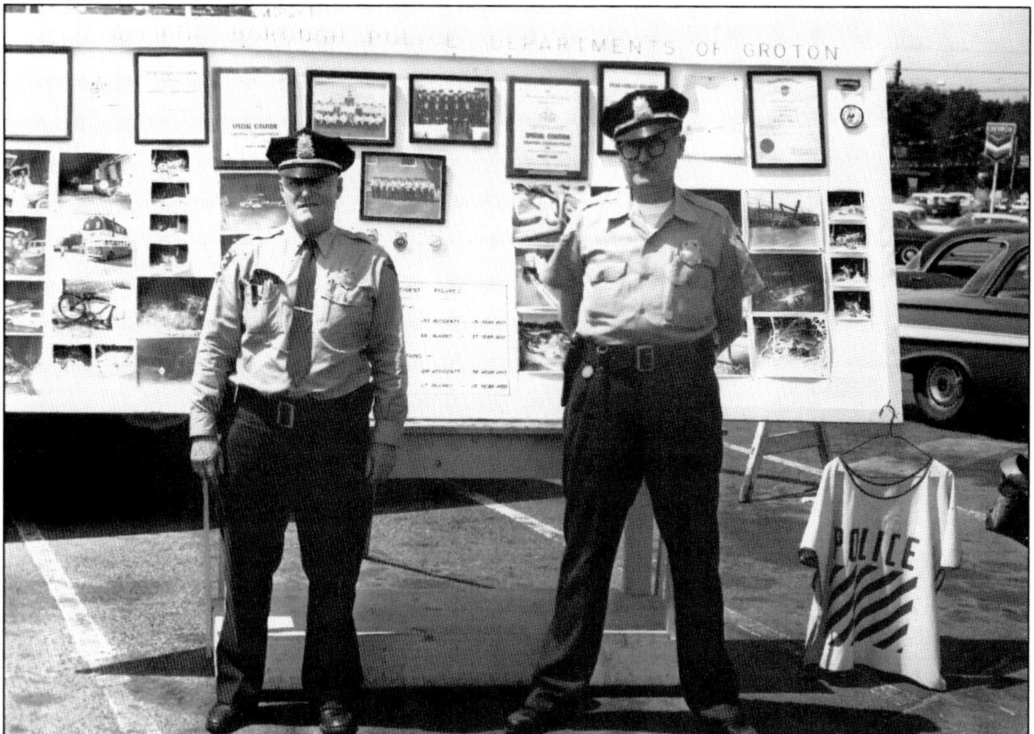
DEPARTMENTS OF GROTON
POLICE

In this c. 1963 photograph, Town of Groton police chief John Scroggins (left) and City of Groton police sergeant John Iverson pose in front of a large display providing the public with information about various police programs and services provided by each of their respective departments. (Town of Groton Police Department.)

Although there is no documented information about the official establishment of the City of Groton Police Department (formerly the Borough of Groton Police Department), archival articles appearing in the *New London Day* newspaper indicate that the Connecticut Legislature passed a law in 1919 to set up the police department. The department employed two patrolmen in 1922, and at that time, the warden of the borough was in charge of the department. According to a July 2015 police study, the department has a staff of 29 officers. (City of Groton Police Department.)

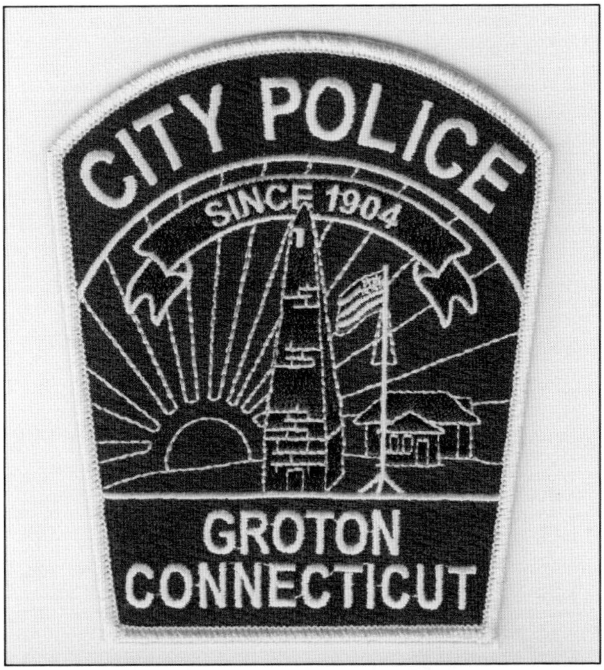

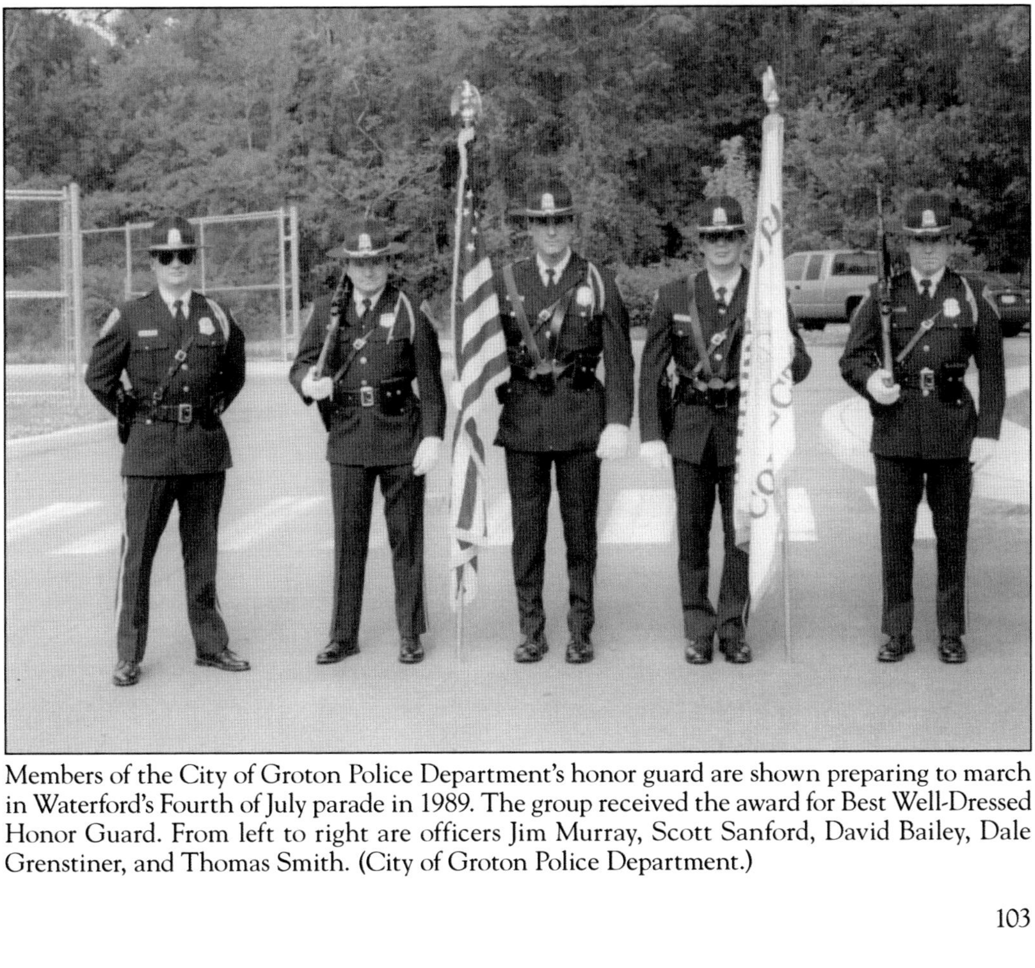

Members of the City of Groton Police Department's honor guard are shown preparing to march in Waterford's Fourth of July parade in 1989. The group received the award for Best Well-Dressed Honor Guard. From left to right are officers Jim Murray, Scott Sanford, David Bailey, Dale Grenstiner, and Thomas Smith. (City of Groton Police Department.)

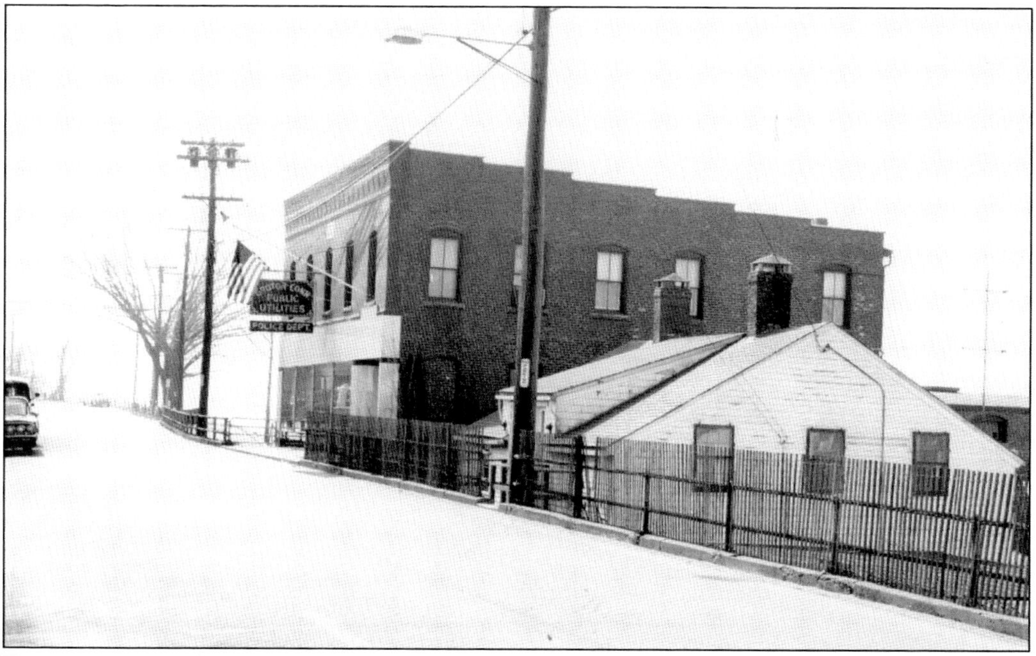

From approximately 1936 through 1966, the Borough of Groton Police Department headquarters and operational spaces were located on the second floor of the former Utilities Department Building on Thames Street, pictured here around 1965. The department ultimately outgrew this limited space and moved to its current location in the City of Groton Municipal Building. (Jim Streeter.)

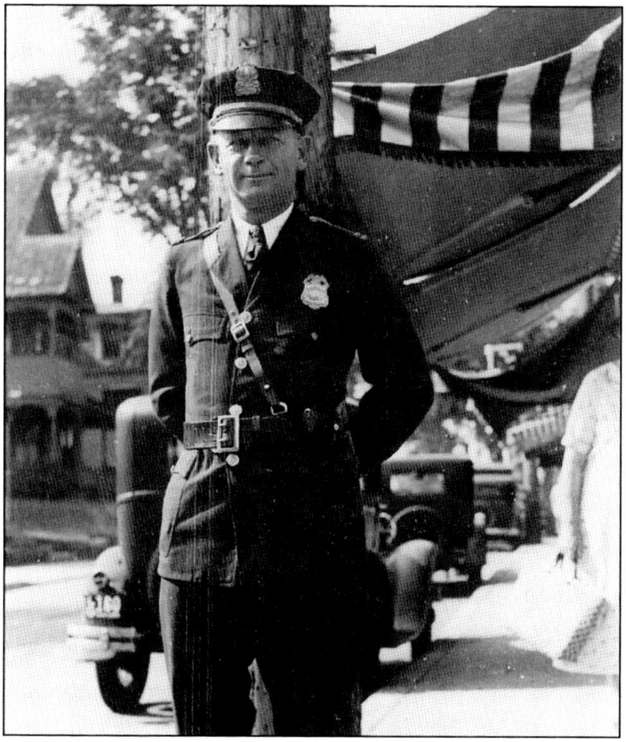

On January 10, 1961, Capt. Bernard Chapman, a 39-year veteran of the Borough of Groton Police Department, died as a result a heart attack while on duty at police headquarters. Captain Chapman joined the department in 1922, when it consisted of two men. He worked his way up through the ranks and was appointed captain in 1931. During his tenure as the ranking officer of the department, the force steadily expanded to a complement of 22 members. (William Hart.)

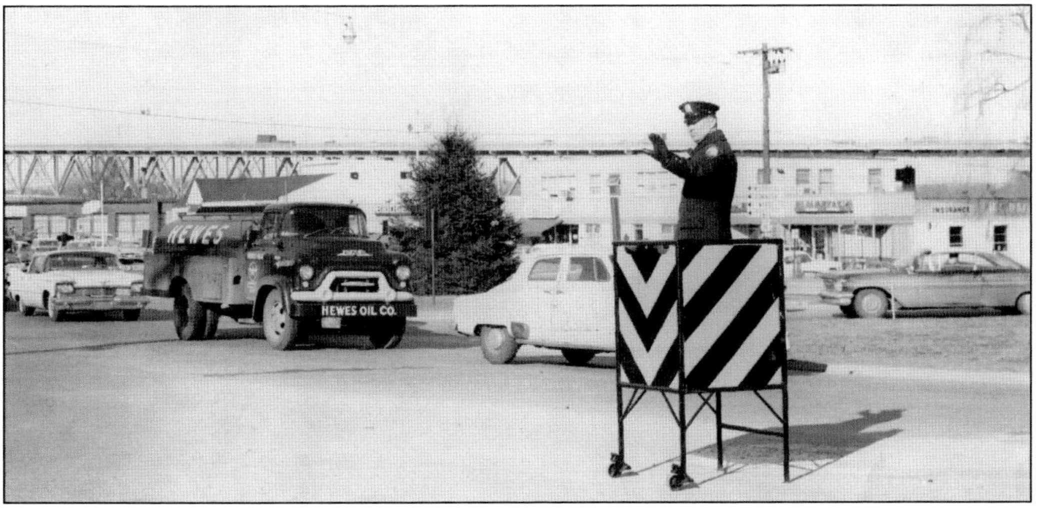

In this c. 1960 photograph, patrolman William Hart of the Borough of Groton Police Department directs traffic from a portable elevated traffic booth at the former rotary (or roundabout) at the intersection of Bridge Street, North Street, Bridge Street Extension, and the Interstate 95 bridge approach. Directing traffic at this intersection was a necessity because of the thousands of vehicles that departed from the Borough of Groton after first shift at Electric Boat, Pfizer, and the Naval Submarine Base New London. Traffic signals installed at this intersection in the 1980s eliminated the need for police to direct traffic here. (William Hart.)

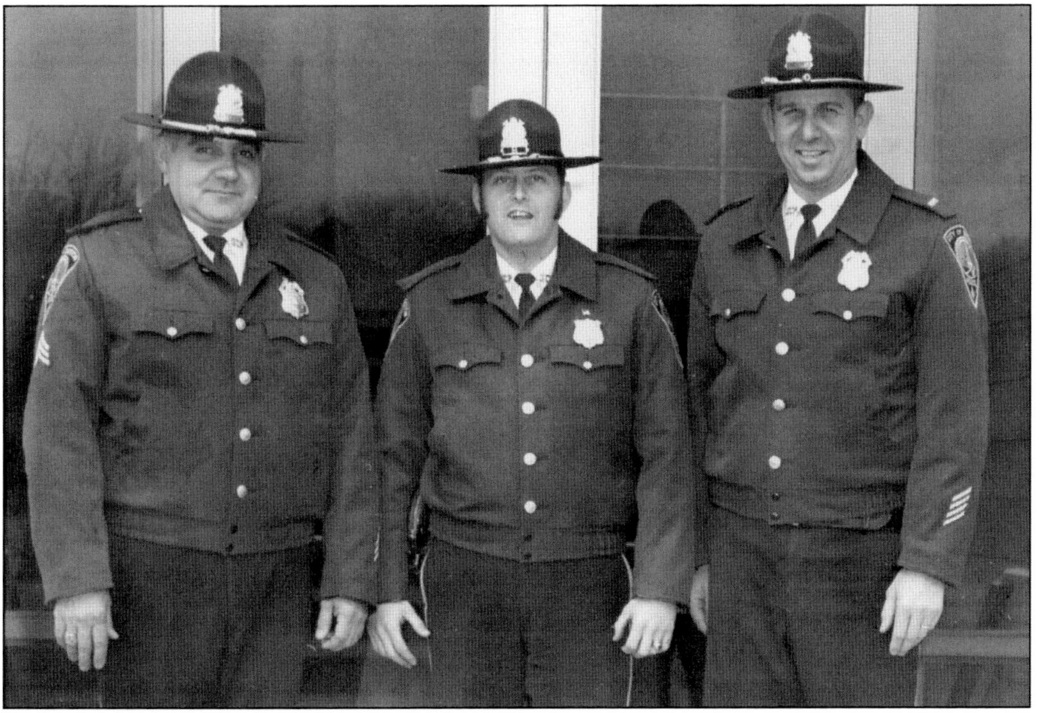

In the early months of 1967, the City of Groton (formerly the Borough of Groton) Police Department changed their uniforms from the standard dark-blue pants and shirt with an eight point–style hat to forest-green pants, white shirts, brown leather accessories, and a ranger-style hat. From left to right are Sgt. Martin Artale, patrolman James Streeter, and Lt. Joseph Sandora. (Jim Streeter.)

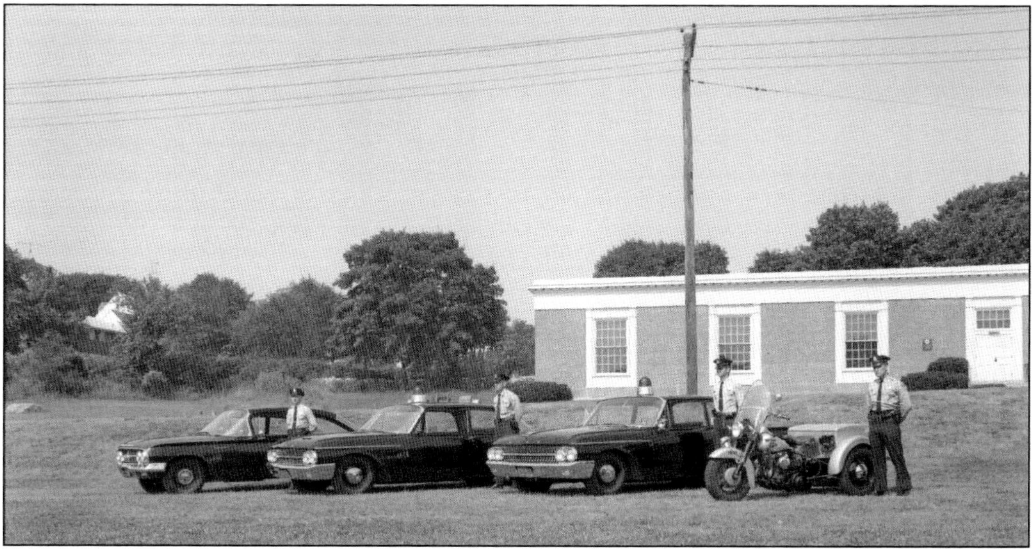

This photograph, taken in the early 1960s, shows the fleet of police vehicles for the Borough of Groton Police Department. Pictured next to the vehicles are, from left to right, patrolmen Roger Fiore, William Hornberger, David White, and David Dunn. (Jim Streeter.)

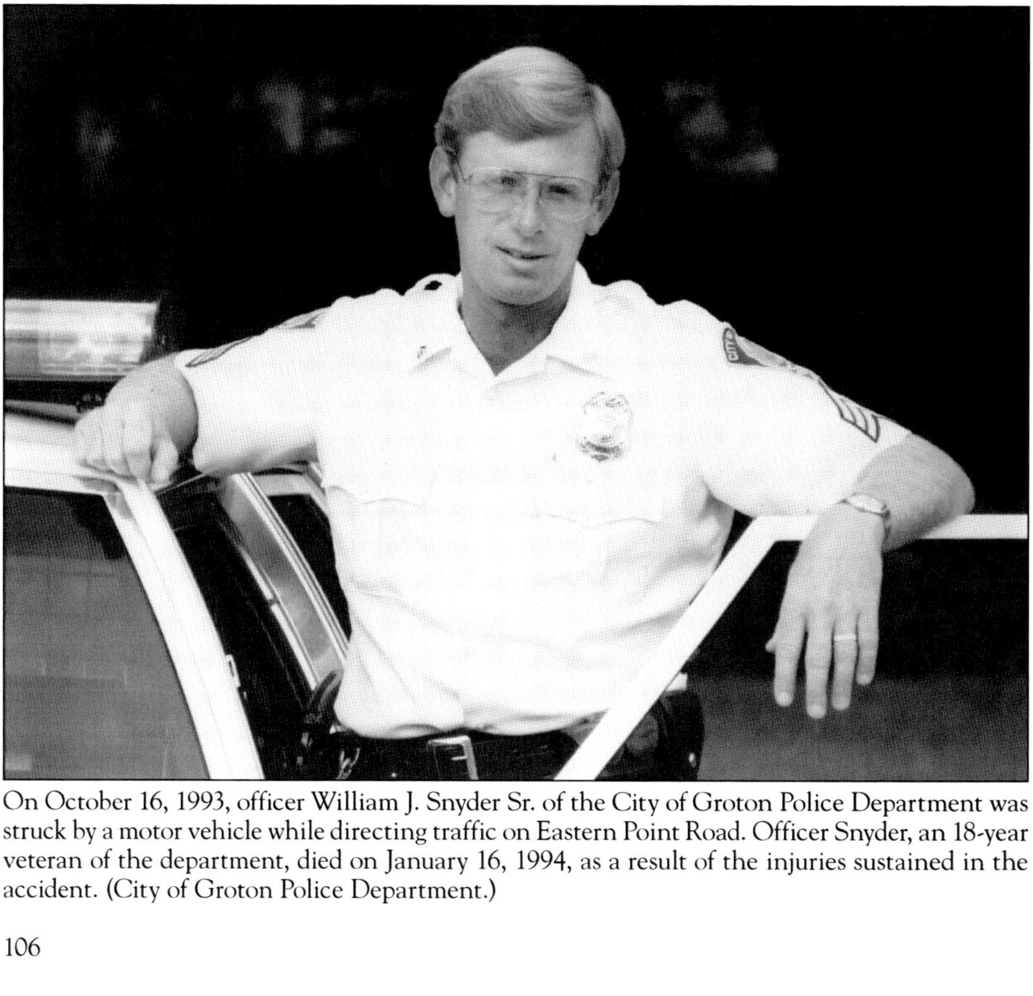

On October 16, 1993, officer William J. Snyder Sr. of the City of Groton Police Department was struck by a motor vehicle while directing traffic on Eastern Point Road. Officer Snyder, an 18-year veteran of the department, died on January 16, 1994, as a result of the injuries sustained in the accident. (City of Groton Police Department.)

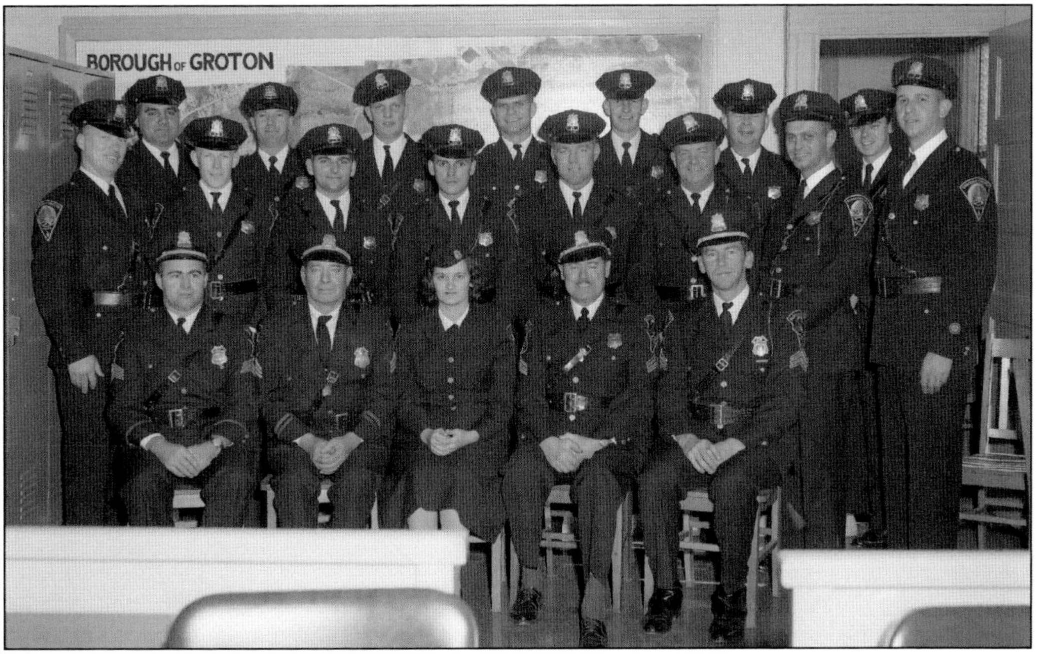

This group photograph of the members of the Borough of Groton (now the City of Groton) Police Department was taken in 1961. From left to right are (first row) Sgt. Timothy Giesing, Sgt. Ira Perkins, policewoman Ann Lackey, Sgt. John Iversen, and Sgt. Benjamin Gillis; (second row) patrolmen William Hart, Wallace Trolan, Roger Fiore, Frank Bailey, Malcolm Lyon, John Dunn, Nicholas DeNoia, and Joseph Sandora; (third row) patrolmen Martin Artale, Blake Rainy, John Gill, David White, John Trolan, Forrester Carberg, and Robert Sharp. (Jim Streeter.)

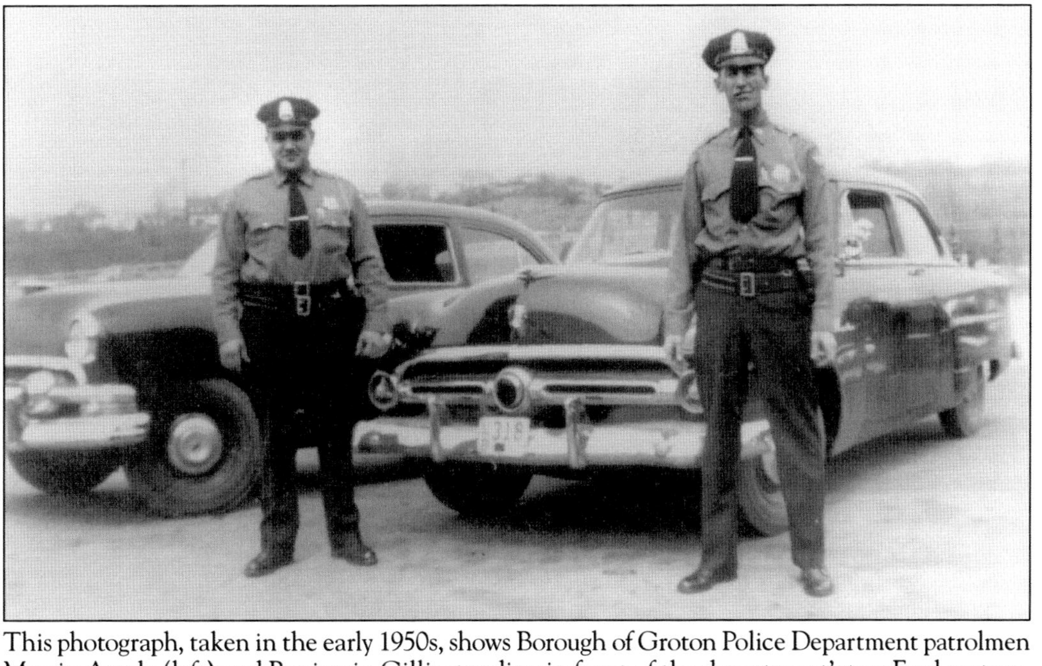

This photograph, taken in the early 1950s, shows Borough of Groton Police Department patrolmen Martin Artale (left) and Benjamin Gillis standing in front of the department's two Ford custom-model police vehicles. (Jim Streeter.)

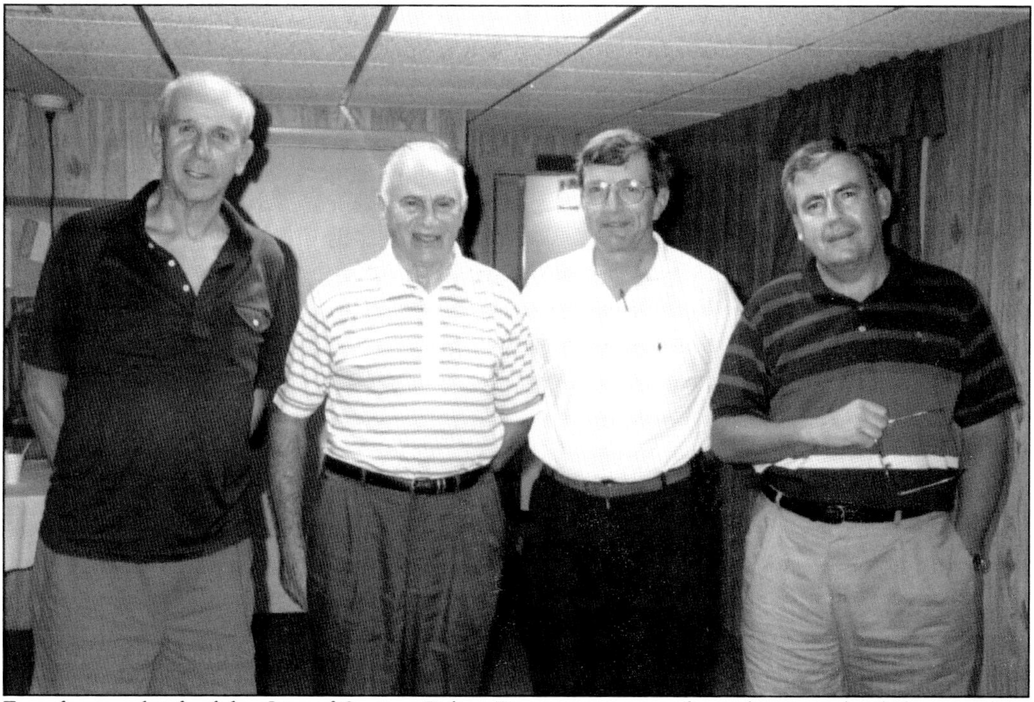

Four former chiefs of the City of Groton Police Department pose for a photograph while attending a gathering for former police officers at the Italian Club in 1990. Pictured here are, from left to right (with their dates of serving as chief in parentheses), Joseph Sandora (1978–1986), Timothy Giesing (1968–1978), Wilfred Blanchette (1990–1998), and Robert Laurie (1986–1990). (Jim Streeter.)

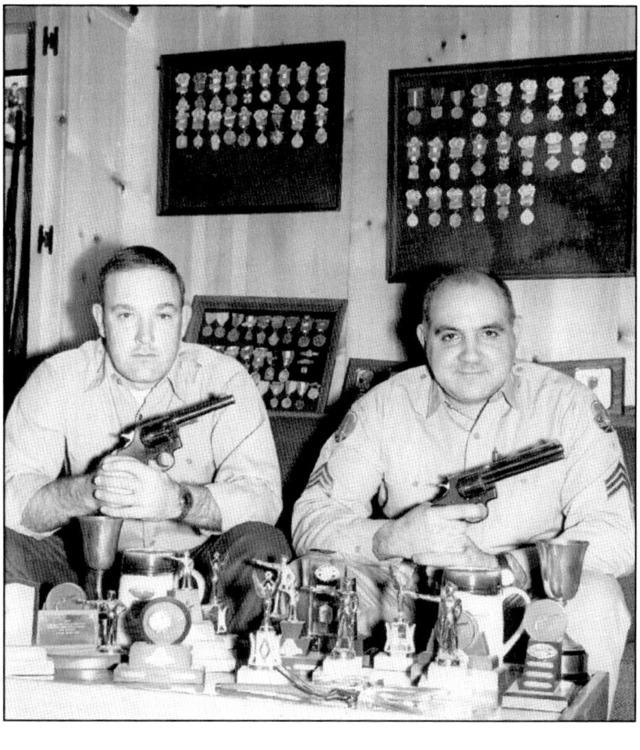

In this photograph from early 1967, patrolman James Sheehan (left) and Sgt. Martin Artale of the City of Groton Police Department proudly display 25 individual and team trophies and 60 medals won by members of the City of Groton Police Department Pistol Team during the preceding six months. The city's pistol team was recognized throughout New England for their excellence in shooting during very competitive police combat matches. (Martin Artale.)

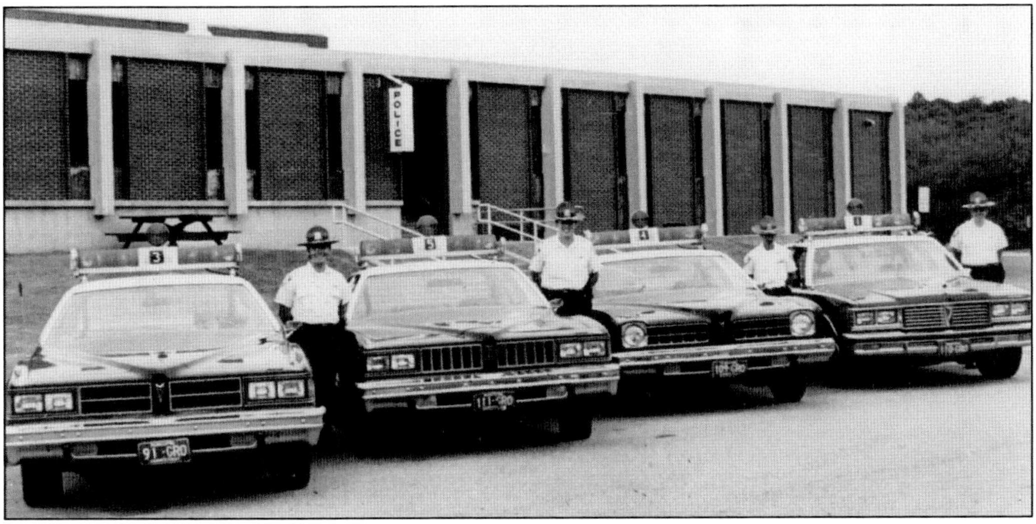

The City of Groton's fleet of police cruisers is pictured outside the department's facilities at the municipal building in 1980. Standing next to the vehicles are, from left to right, patrolmen Dennis Campagna, Dale Grenstiner, William Stewart, and Frank Slavinski. (Dale Grenstiner.)

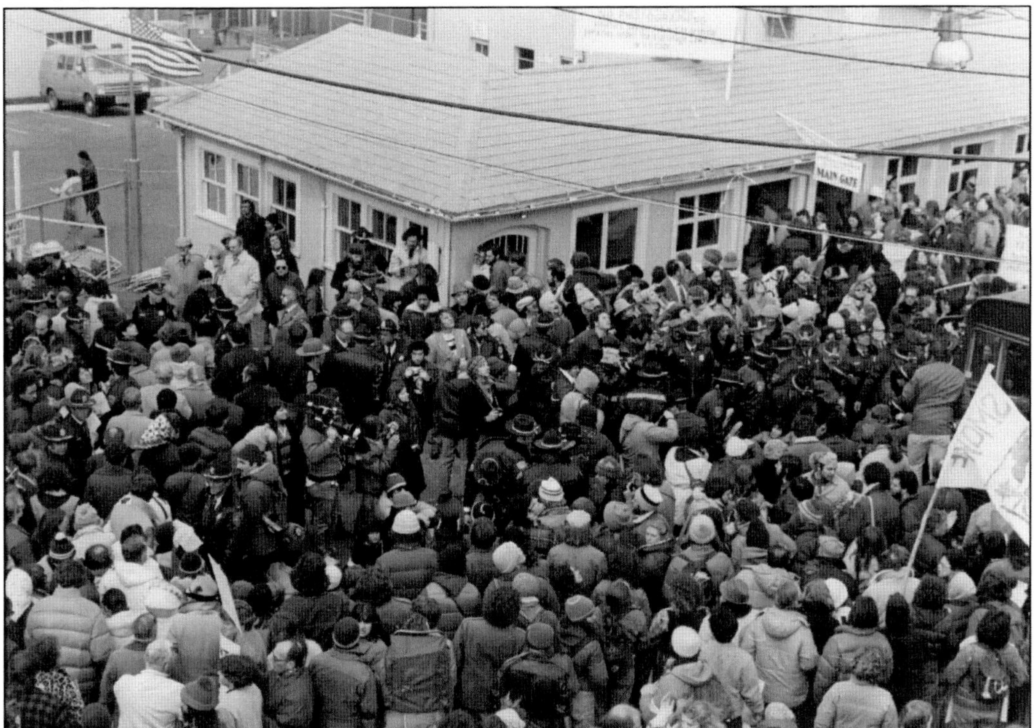

On April 7, 1979, one of the largest antinuclear protests in the country took place outside the gates of Electric Boat in Groton during the launching ceremony for the USS *Ohio*, the first Trident-class missile submarine. The number of protesters exceeded 3,000, and more than 300 of those individuals were arrested for various misdemeanor violations. Here, police officers from both the City of Groton and Town of Groton Police Departments are shown controlling protest activities and carrying several protesters to police containment vehicles. (Jim Streeter.)

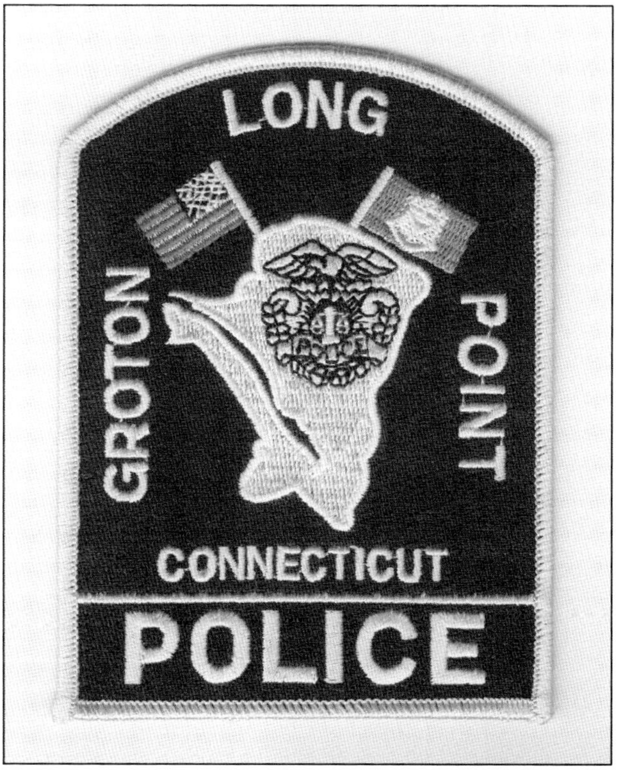

As best as can be determined, the beginning of the Groton Long Point Police Department can be traced back to 1927, when Charles Yering was appointed as a special policeman to enforce various regulations that applied to the Groton Long Point Association proper. In 1964, the association purchased its first police vehicle. Prior to this, Groton Long Point police officers used their own vehicles to patrol and respond to incidents. Today, the association maintains their own dedicated police department, which consists of five sworn officers (including the chief) and four part-time officers. (Groton Long Point Association.)

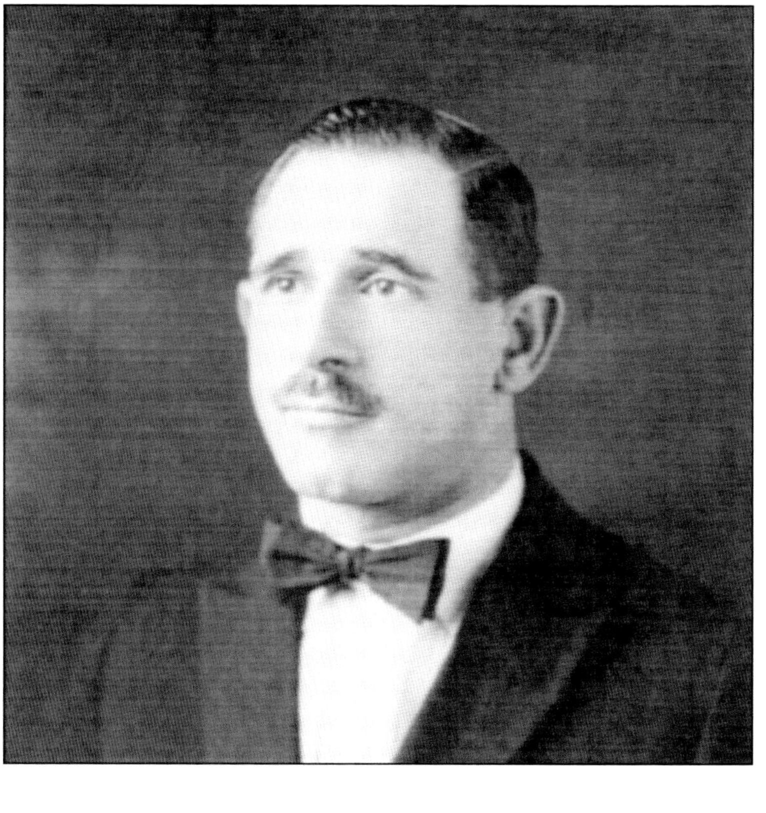

On June 16, 1959, Chief Chares E. Yering, a 32-year veteran of the Groton Long Point Police Department, died as a result a heart attack he suffered while performing patrol duties at Groton Long Point. Yering was appointed as Long Point's first special patrolman in 1927. (Thomas Migliaccio Jr.)

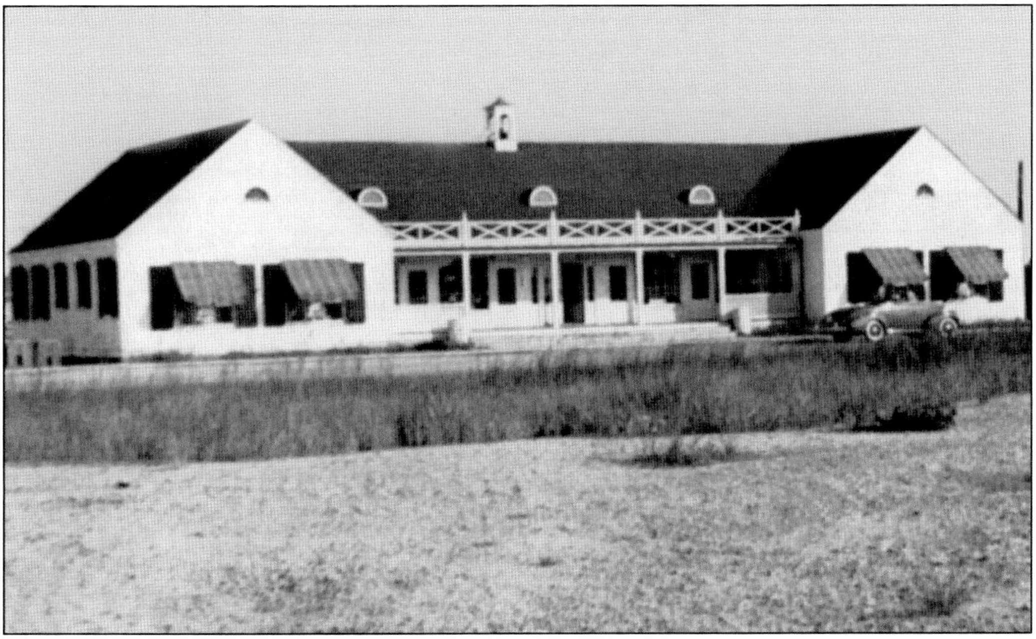

Beginning in April 1985, the Groton Long Point Police Department maintained office spaces at the newly renovated Groton Long Point Association's Casino building. The department remained here until 1990, when they moved to new spaces above the association's fire department on Atlantic Street. This c. 1950 photograph shows the front of the Casino. (Jim Streeter.)

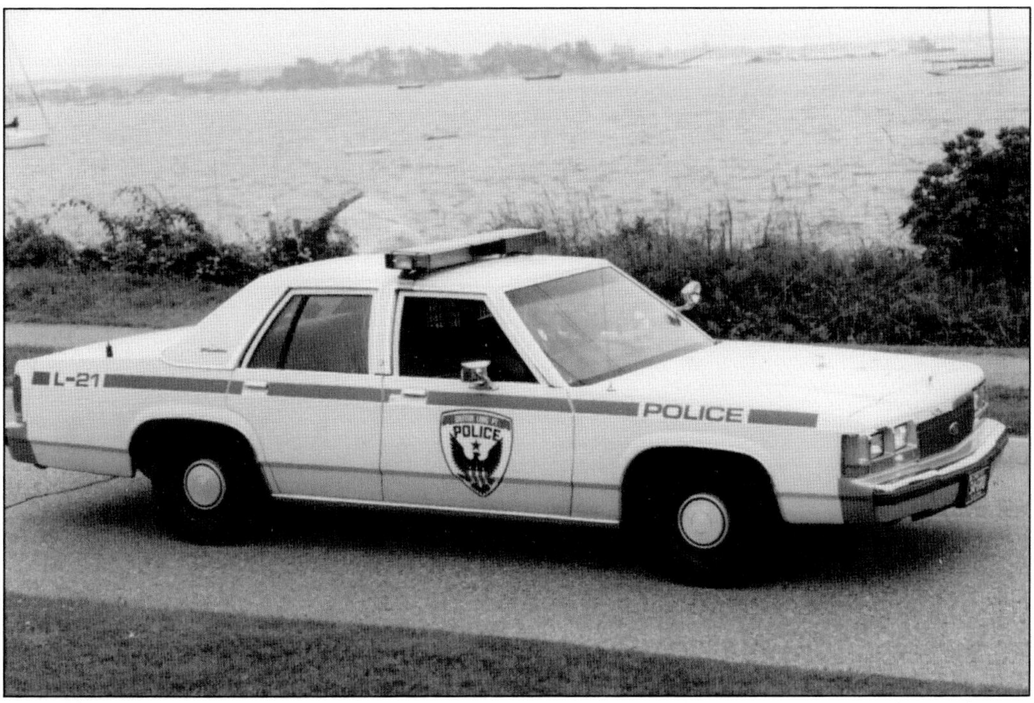

This patrol vehicle from the Groton Long Point Association Police Department is shown during the association's annual Fourth of July parade in 1992. Members of the police department use the vehicle to patrol the Groton Long Point community. (Groton Long Point Association.)

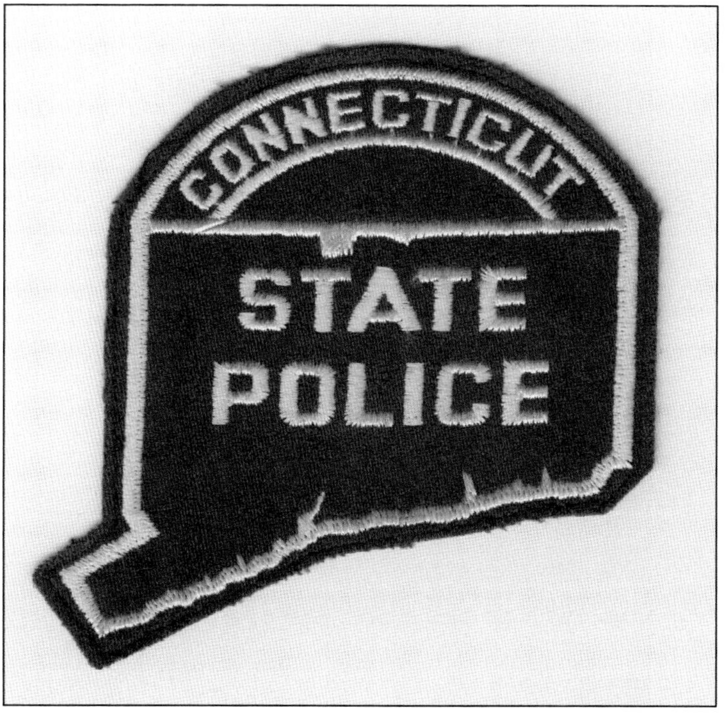

From 1923 through 1973, the Connecticut State Police had a presence in Groton. Although state troopers were mainly responsible for enforcement of Connecticut motor vehicle laws, they have authority to enforce criminal laws throughout the state. Local police departments, including those in Groton, often did not have the staff or resources, such as equipment and training, to conduct investigations involving major criminal offenses or activities. Thus, state police would assume the responsibility of overseeing these matters. (Jim Streeter.)

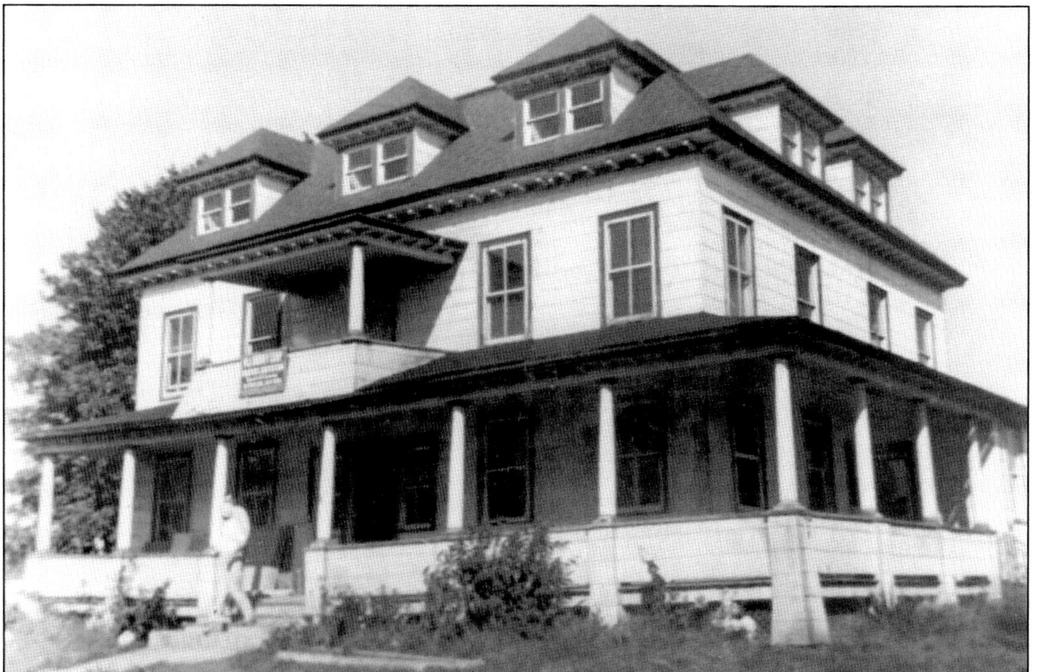

In 1923, the state police established Station No. 6 in what was once a privately owned house on Eastern Point Road in Groton. Initially, only one or two troopers manned the station. Shortly after the station went into operation, a class of 37 police recruits reported to this station for their three-week police training. This photograph was taken around 1935. (Jim Streeter.)

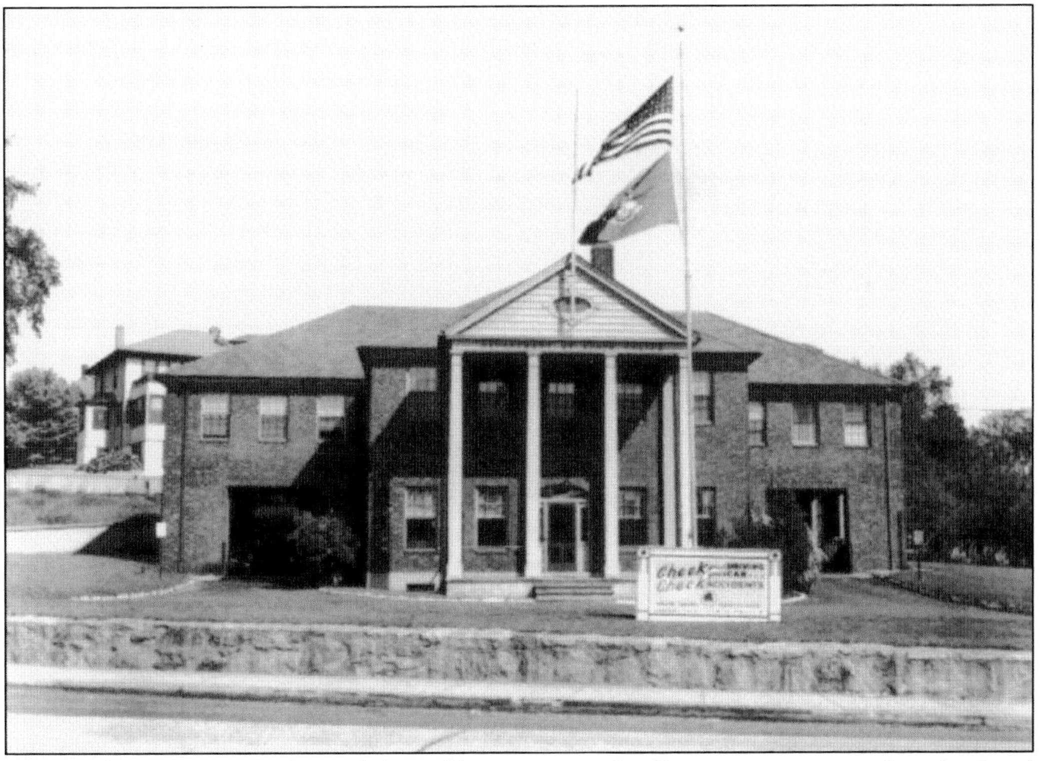

In 1931, the Connecticut General Assembly appropriated sufficient money to purchase land and build a new two-story brick station at the intersection of Bridge Street and Thames Street in Groton. After this building was completed, the station moved here from its former location on Eastern Point Road. Beginning in 1939, state police facilities were referred to as barracks rather than stations. The police barracks in Groton was named Troop E. (Jim Streeter.)

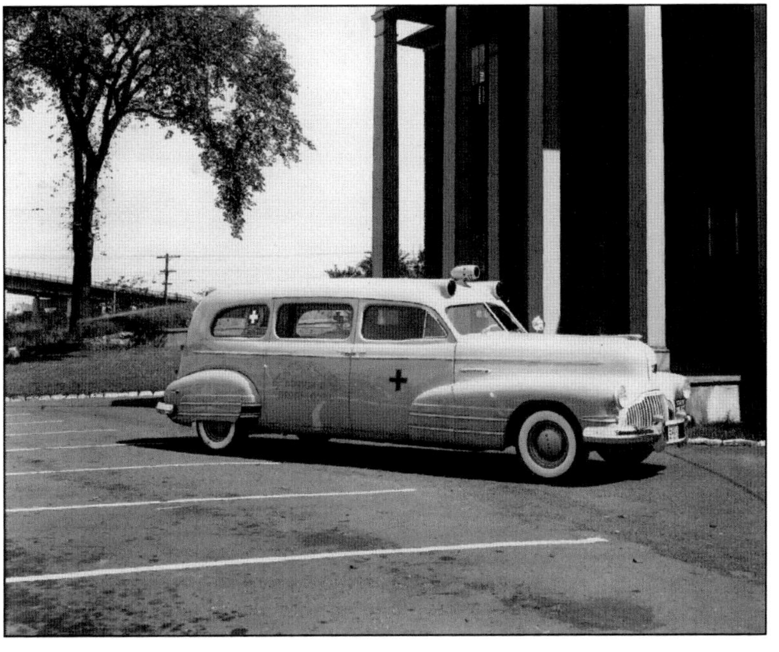

In 1942, Mary Harkness donated an ambulance to the state police station in Groton. The "Harkness Ambulance" (pictured here around 1945) proved its value hundreds of times during emergencies, particularly when covering points from east of the Connecticut River to the border of Rhode Island. (Jim Streeter.)

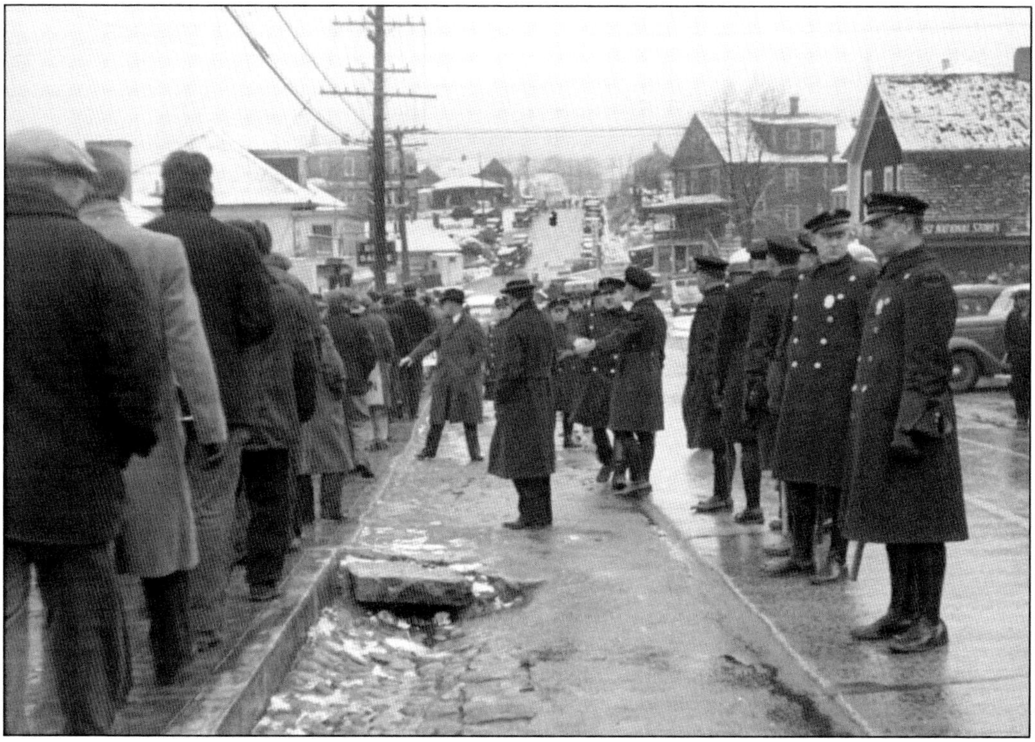

Troopers from the Groton State Police station are shown monitoring strikers at Electric Boat in 1937. Due to limited local manpower, state police would often oversee major incidents and labor strikes that occurred throughout the state. (Jim Streeter.)

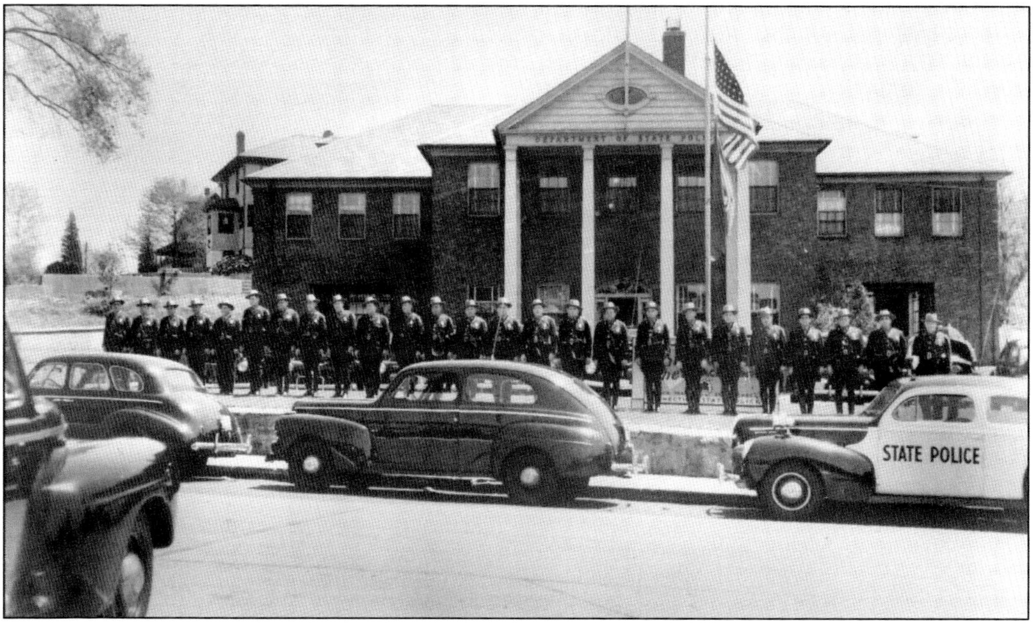

State troopers assigned to Troop E in Groton pose in front of their barracks at the intersection of Bridge and Thames Streets in the late 1940s. Also pictured are the vehicles used by the troopers. (Jim Streeter.)

Four

Ambulances and Other Support Services

In addition to the services provided by the numerous fire and police departments in Groton, other very important and necessary emergency services are provided by other agencies.

The Groton Ambulance Association, Inc., and the Mystic River Ambulance Association, Inc., provide high-quality emergency medical service care and emergency medical transportation. Both associations are staffed with paid and volunteer professionals.

The Lawrence + Memorial Hospital paramedics provide another important service in Groton and Mystic. These highly trained individuals respond to medical emergencies and provide advanced life support to sick and injured people at their homes or at the scene of an accident.

Another group that provides an all-important service to the various emergency service departments is the Groton Emergency Dispatch Center. The center is operated around the clock by certified emergency telephone dispatchers who are responsible for the receipt and transmission of emergency communications and directing the response of emergency services throughout all of Groton. The dispatchers in this center perform their tasks 24 hours per day, 365 days per year, and are considered by some to be the "first responders" to all calls.

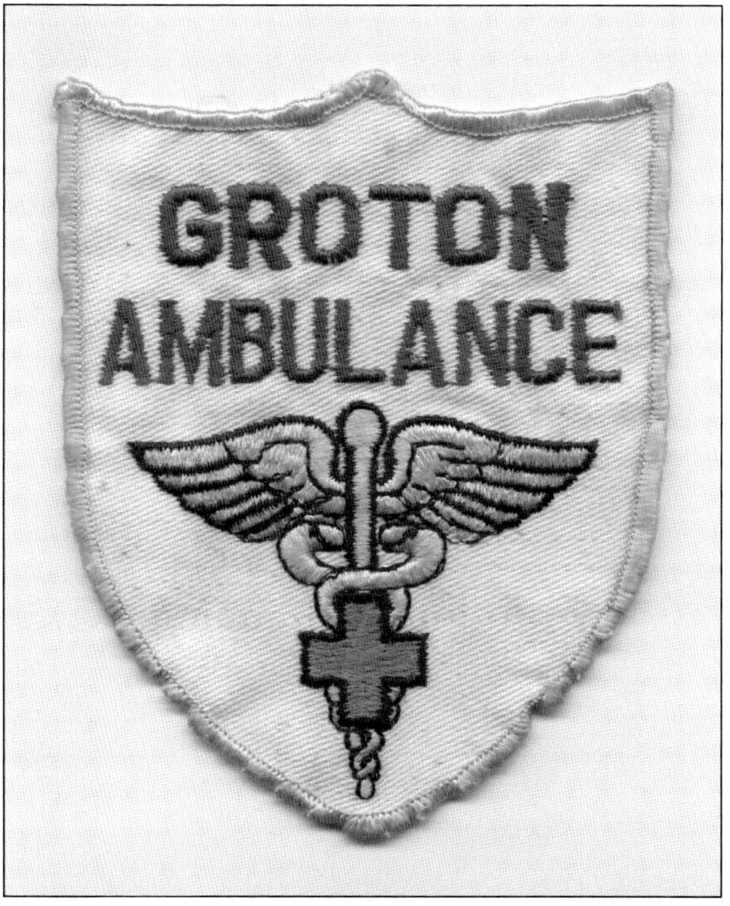

Groton Ambulance Service, Inc., started in April 1947. It became Groton Ambulance Association when it was chartered by the state on December 7, 1954. The service's first facility was located at the Trumbull Airport and later moved to a new building on Tower Avenue. The association is now located in a modern building on Newtown Road. (Groton Ambulance Association.)

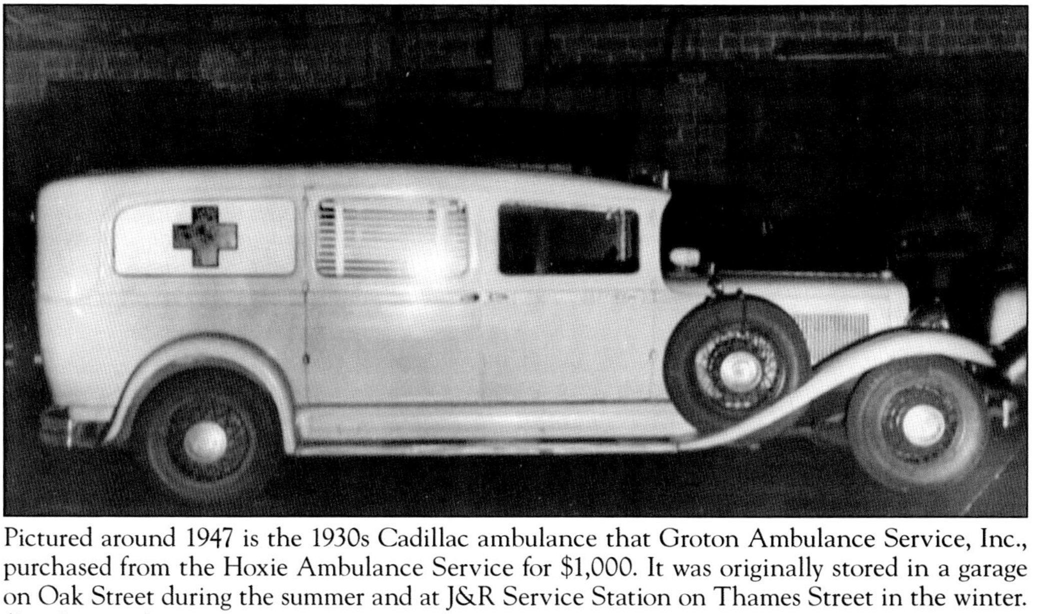

Pictured around 1947 is the 1930s Cadillac ambulance that Groton Ambulance Service, Inc., purchased from the Hoxie Ambulance Service for $1,000. It was originally stored in a garage on Oak Street during the summer and at J&R Service Station on Thames Street in the winter. (Jim Streeter.)

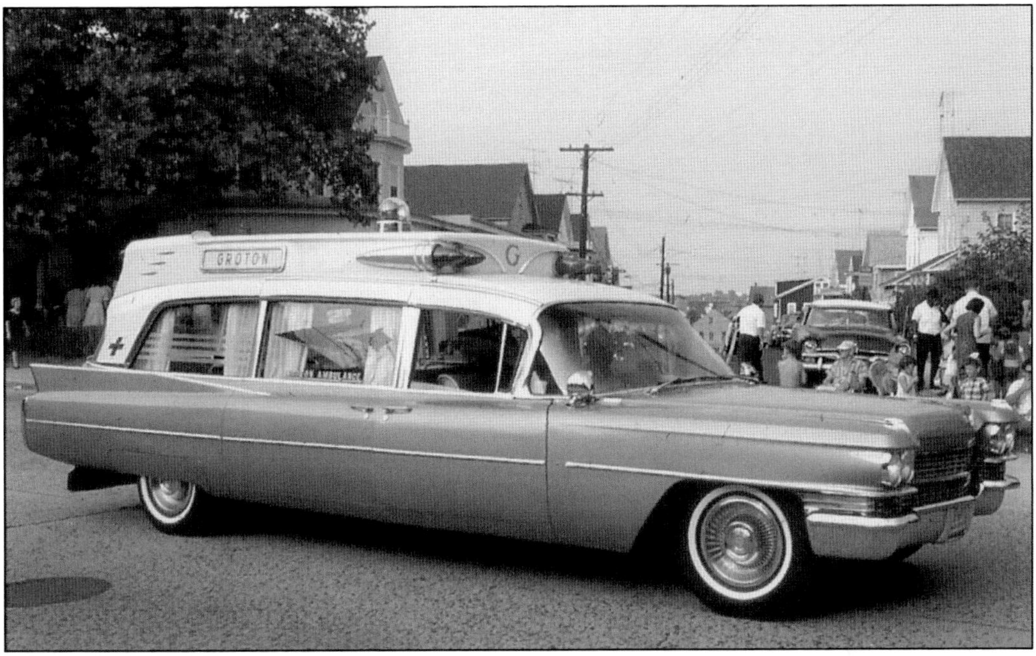

Groton Ambulance Association's 1962 Cadillac paraded down Montauk Avenue during New London's State Firemen's Convention in 1966. When this vehicle was purchased, the lending bank required the association's members to put up their own homes as collateral to sign for the loan. (Pioneer Hose Company.)

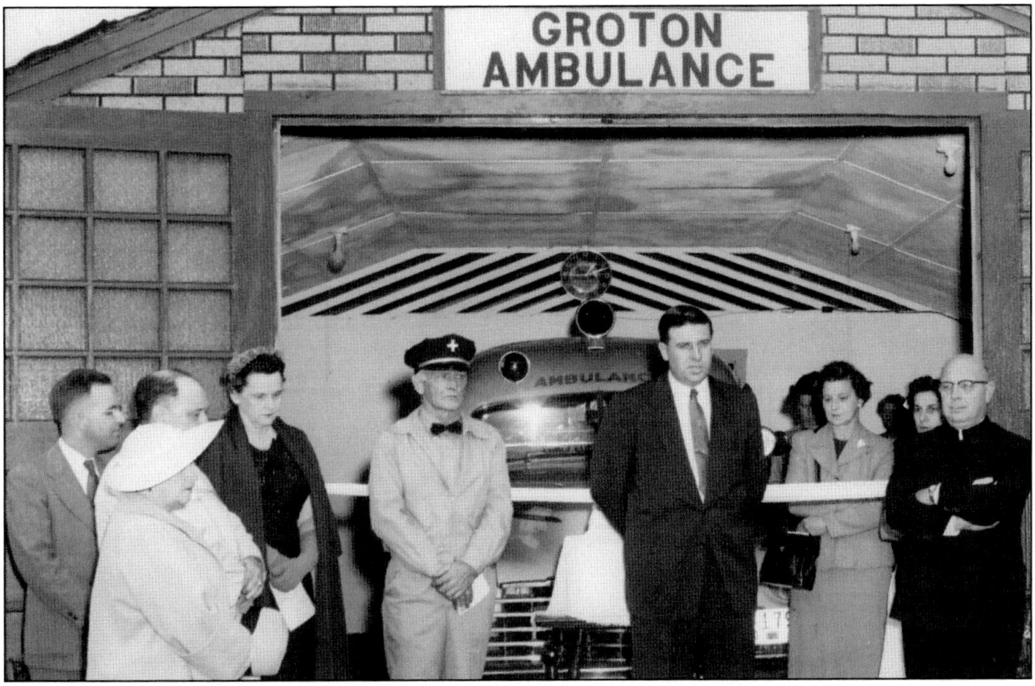

On June 11, 1955, at a gathering of about 200 people, the Groton Ambulance Association dedicated their new building, which was donated to them, at the Trumbull Airport. President Newton Maynard (in uniform) cut the silver ribbon at the event. (Groton Ambulance Association.)

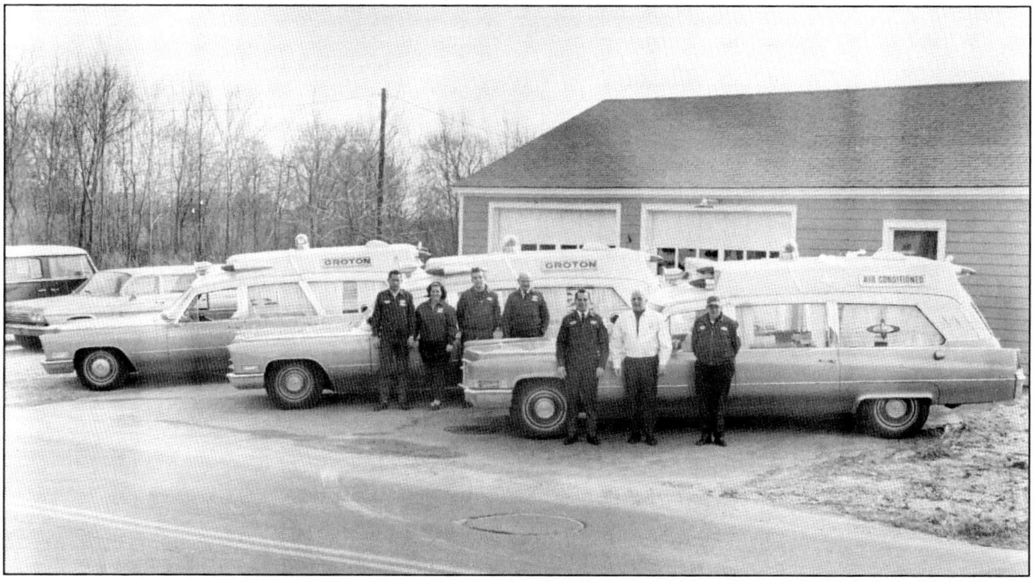

Groton Ambulance's fleet of Cadillacs sits in front of their Tower Avenue quarters with some unidentified association members. The ambulances were painted gold and white because Groton Ambulance president Emil Eckholme believed the color would represent class and prestige. (Groton Ambulance Association.)

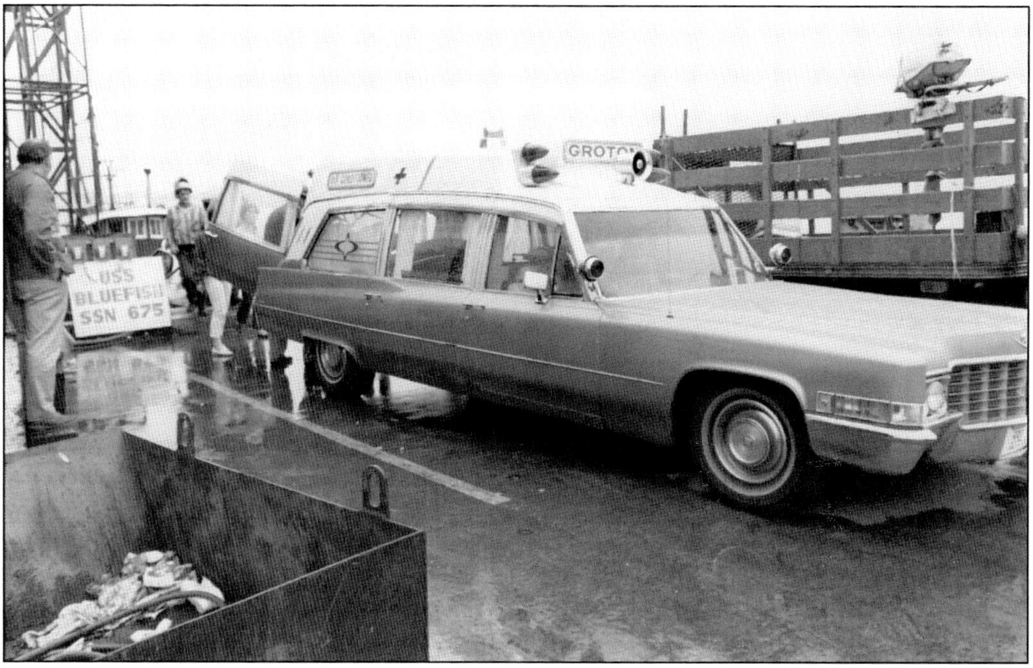

In this c. 1970 photograph, a patient on a litter is being removed from a Groton Ambulance Association ambulance at the Electric Boat shipyard in Groton before being placed on a tugboat and transported across the Thames River to New London, where another ambulance would then take the patient to the Lawrence + Memorial Hospital. This method of transporting patients to the hospital in New London was necessary when there was a traffic tie-up on the vehicle bridge that crosses the river. (Groton Ambulance Association.)

Unfortunately, accidents do occur. Groton Ambulance's 1958 Cadillac is pictured here after it hit a truck in New London on Wednesday, July 29, 1964. Fortunately, no one was injured in the collision, and the ambulance was not transporting a patient. There was considerable damage to the ambulance but only minor damage to the truck. (Groton Ambulance Association.)

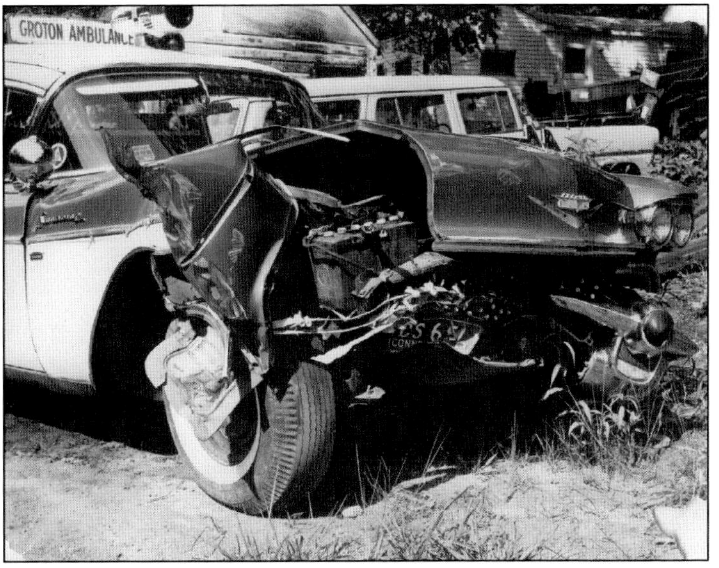

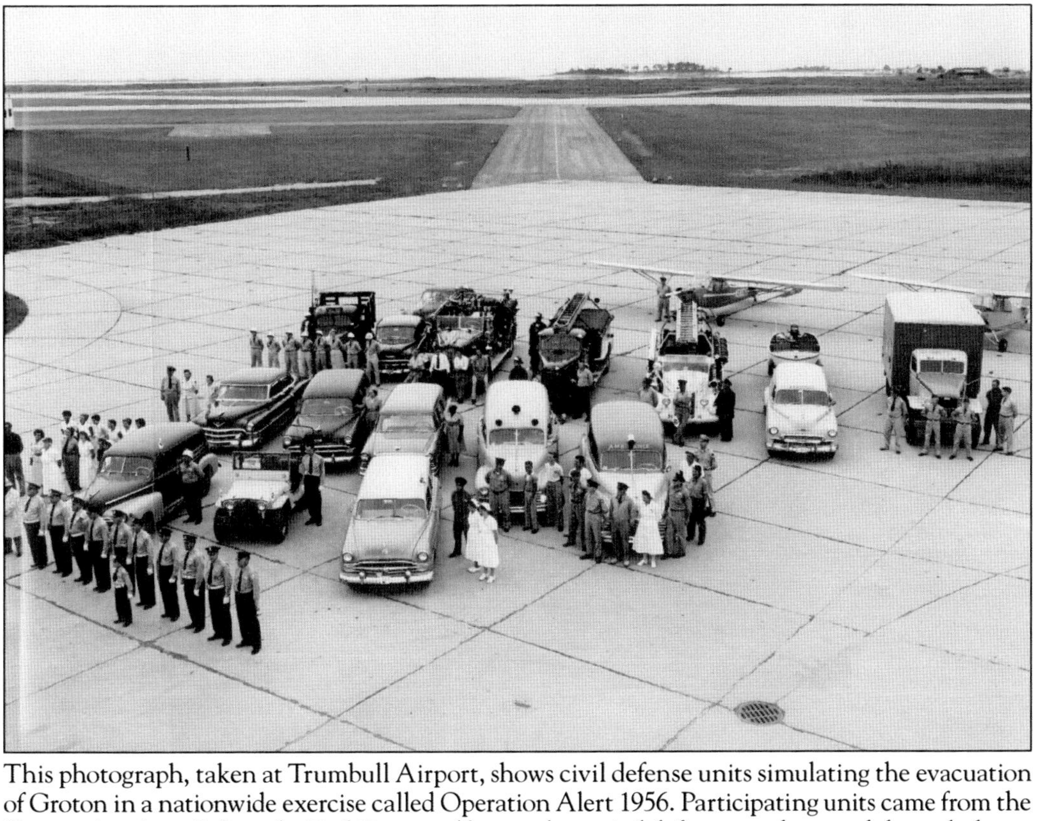

This photograph, taken at Trumbull Airport, shows civil defense units simulating the evacuation of Groton in a nationwide exercise called Operation Alert 1956. Participating units came from the Groton Auxiliary Police, the Red Cross, welfare workers, civil defense wardens, and the ambulance rescue and medical unit. Fire apparatuses from the Borough of Groton, Center Groton, and Poquonnock Bridge—along with aircraft from the Auxiliary Police, Air and Maritime Operations, and Civil Air Patrol—were also on-site. (Jim Streeter.)

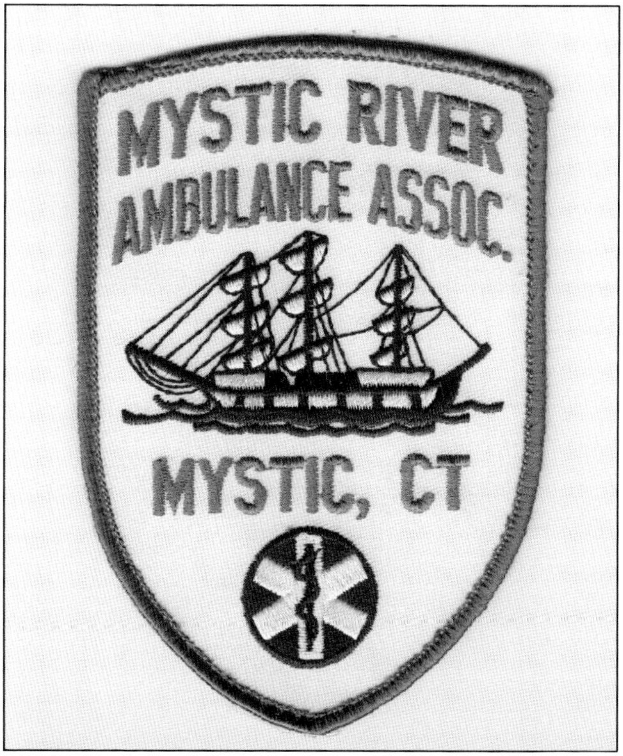

The roots of the Mystic River Ambulance Association go back to April 8, 1945, when the B.F. Hoxie Engine Company approved $550 to buy a 1931 hearse and convert it into an ambulance, which would cost another $100. That vehicle was replaced with a new ambulance in March 1947. The Hoxies announced plans to end ambulance service in 1981; it was then that the Mystic River Ambulance Association began. (Mystic River Ambulance Association.)

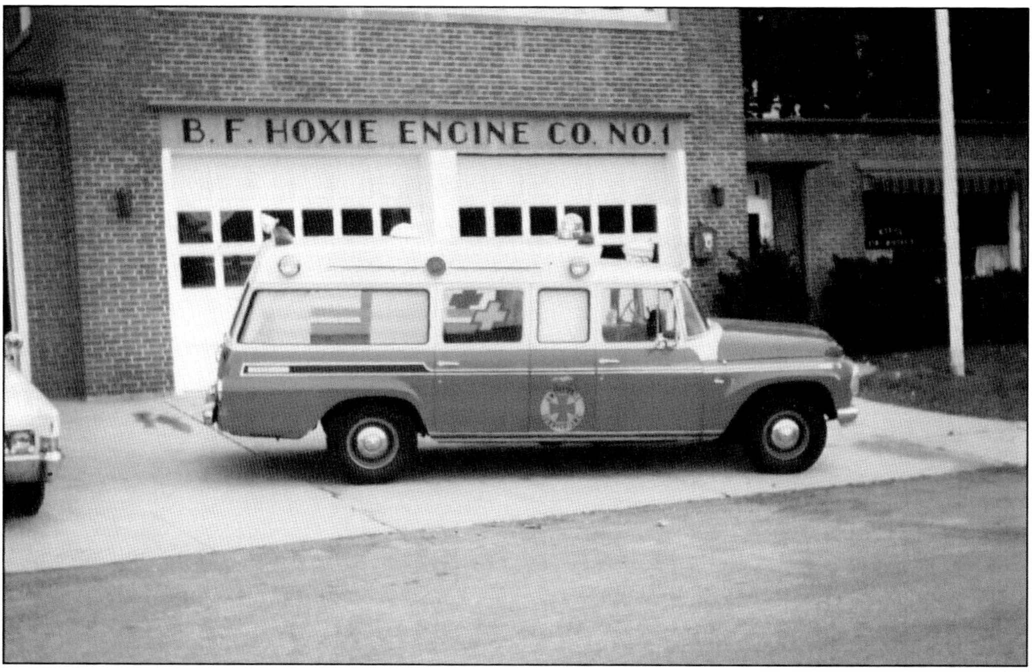

In August 1968, the B.F. Hoxie Engine Company, which was responsible for ambulance service in the Mystic area, took delivery of this new International Harvester panel ambulance, which cost $10,000. In 1981, the Hoxies discontinued providing ambulance service in Mystic; subsequently, the Mystic River Ambulance Association was established. (Mystic River Ambulance Association.)

The Hoxies purchased this Dodge ambulance with a trade-in at a cost of $17,000 in 1975. This new style of van had considerably more room in the patient compartment, but its motion could not compare to the Cadillac's smooth ride. (Mystic River Ambulance Association.)

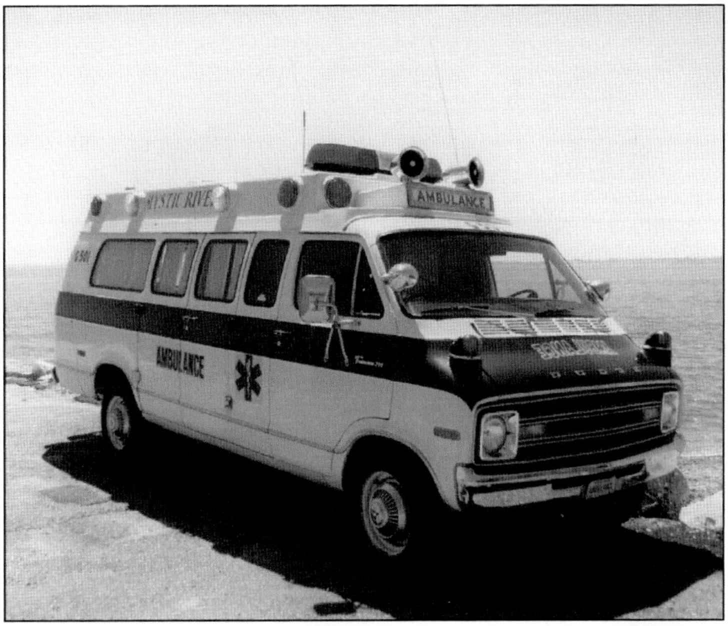

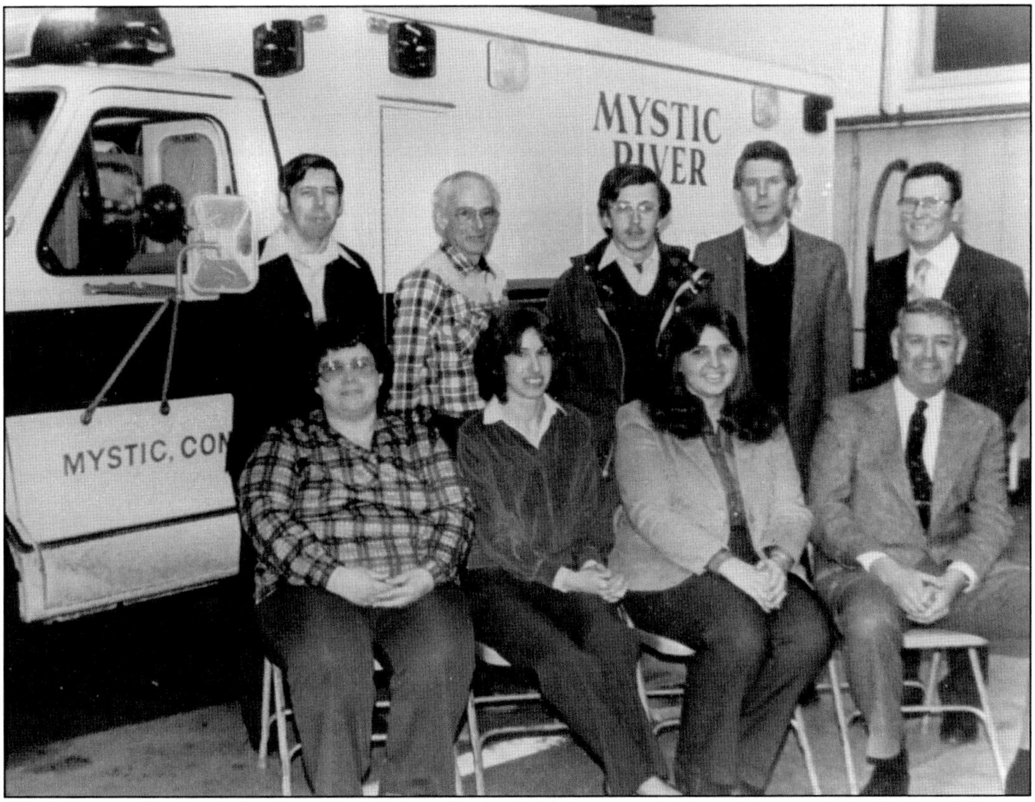

The founding members of the Mystic River Ambulance Association pictured here in the early 1980s are, from left to right, (first row) Sue May, Jane Cannon, Cathy Fox, and Charlie Maxon; (second row) Robert Sylvestre, Charlie Main, Frank Brewer, Ed Hanks, and George Fargo. (Mystic River Ambulance Association.)

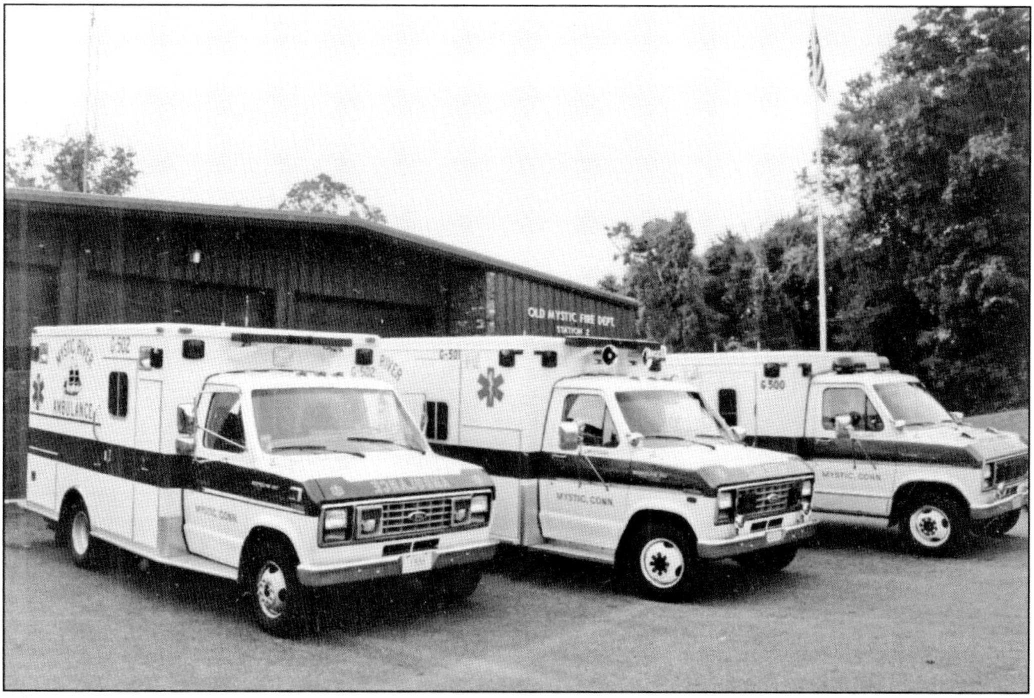

This c. 1991 photograph was taken prior to the Mystic River Ambulance Association having its own quarters. The ambulance fleet is parked in front of the first Old Mystic Fire Department fire station on Cow Hill Road. At that time, one ambulance was kept here, a second was kept at the B.F. Hoxie station on Cottrell Street, and a third—a spare—was kept at the Electric Boat Fire Department in the City of Groton. (Mystic River Ambulance Association.)

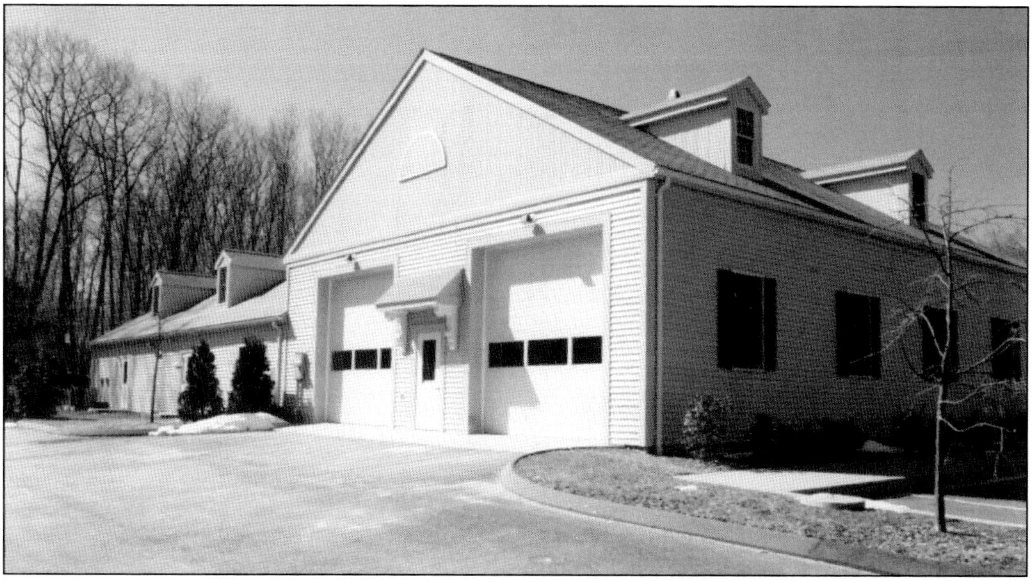

In 1991, Mystic residents initiated a fundraising drive to collect money to build new facilities to house the Mystic River Ambulance Association's vehicles and equipment. The campaign was successful, and in January 1993, the association moved to these new facilities at the intersection of Allyn Street and Sandy Hollow Road. (Mystic River Ambulance Association.)

After two years of planning, Lawrence + Memorial Hospital initiated a paramedic response program on March 19, 1988. It was a new concept for the area, but the community would soon recognize its worth. Since the beginning, the Lawrence + Memorial paramedics team has taken many lifesaving actions. Eventually, Lawrence + Memorial Hospital Paramedics assigned a vehicle to each side of the Thames River. (Lawrence + Memorial Hospital Paramedics.)

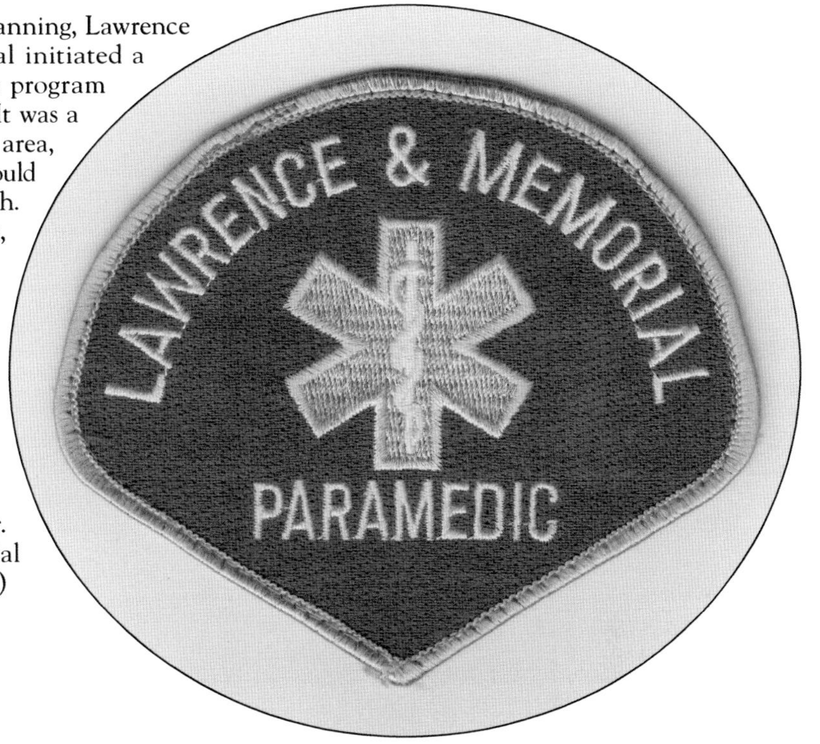

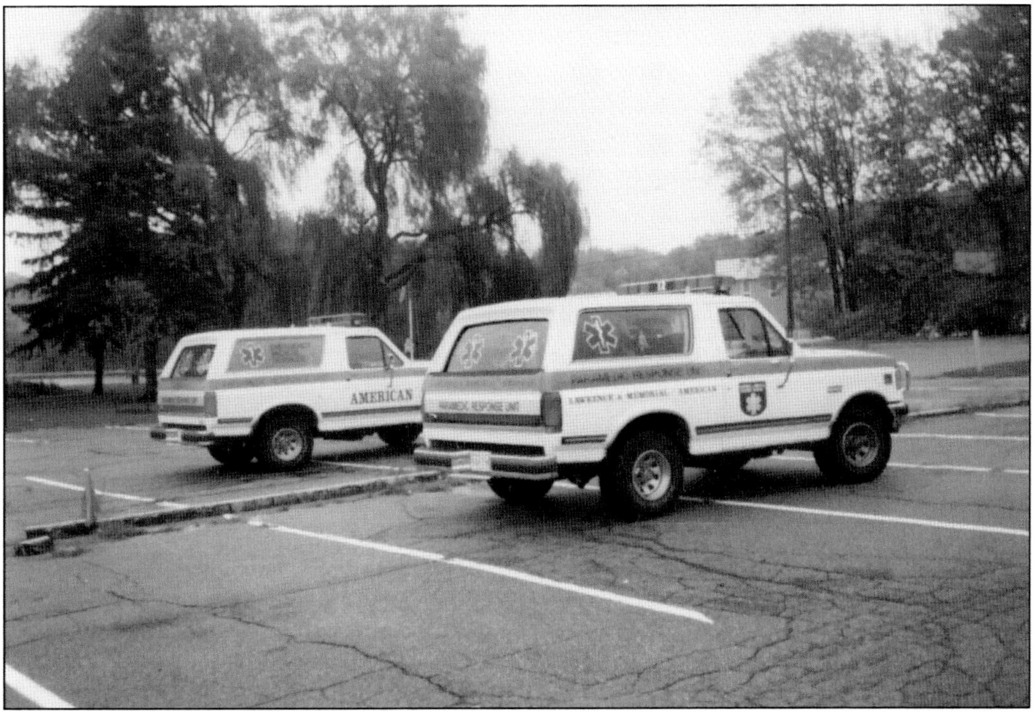

Pictured here around 1990 are two of Lawrence + Memorial's first intercept vehicles. These Ford Broncos were modeled after those used by American Ambulance in Norwich. (Submarine Base New London Fire Department.)

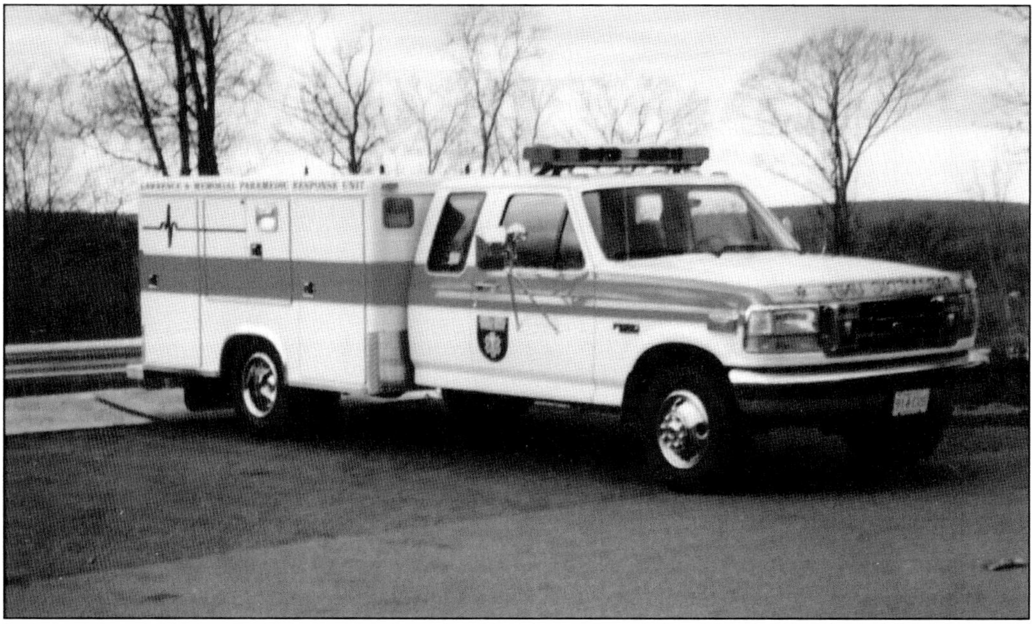

In the 1990s, Lawrence + Memorial Hospital Paramedics purchased larger trucks to facilitate carrying more equipment. Refrigerated compartments were installed in these vehicles to preserve medicine. When dispatched, medics would meet the ambulance at the scene of a call or while en route to the hospital and render care as needed. (Lawrence + Memorial Hospital Paramedics.)

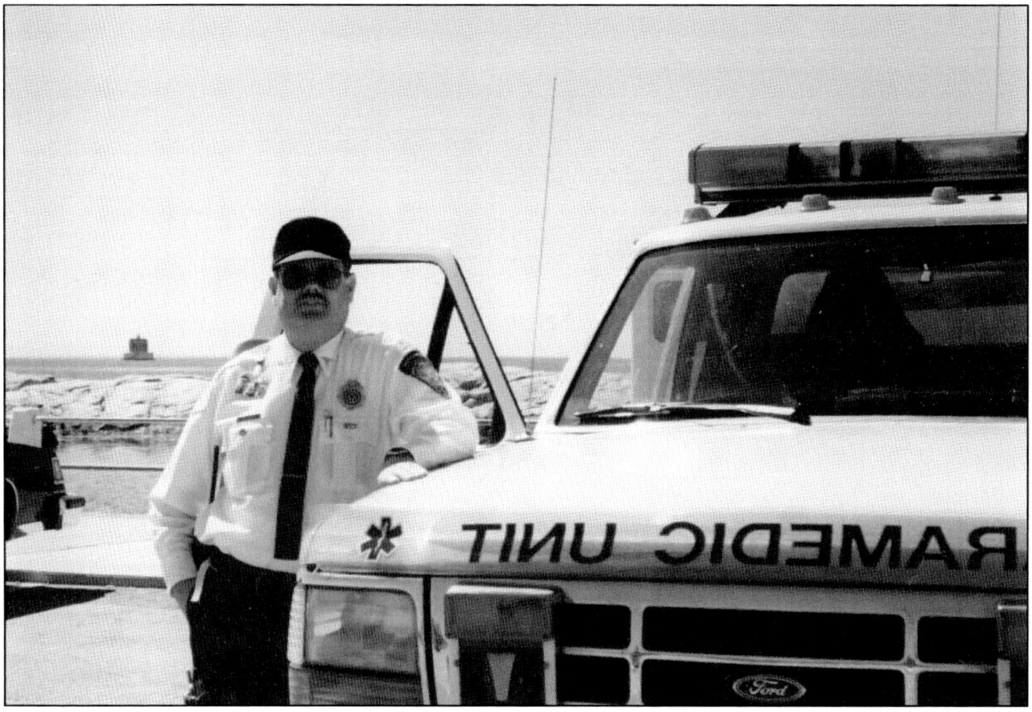

Lawrence + Memorial Hospital paramedic Don Hall stands at the ready with his intercept vehicle in Groton. The medics service an area of over 300 square miles and utilize a staff of eight full-time medics and fifteen part-time employees. (Lawrence + Memorial Hospital Paramedics.)

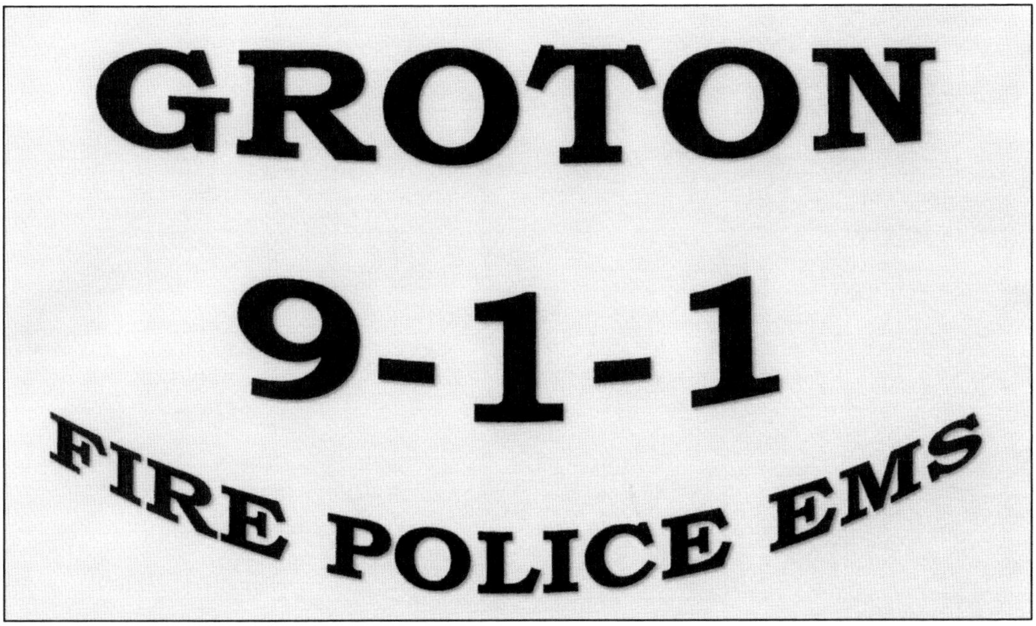

Until 1981, Groton's fire departments were predominantly self-dispatched, and the ambulance association used an answering service. That year, the group decided to install a 911 system and consolidate as the Groton Emergency Communications Center, better known by fire departments and ambulances as Groton Fire Alarm. (Groton Emergency Communications Center.)

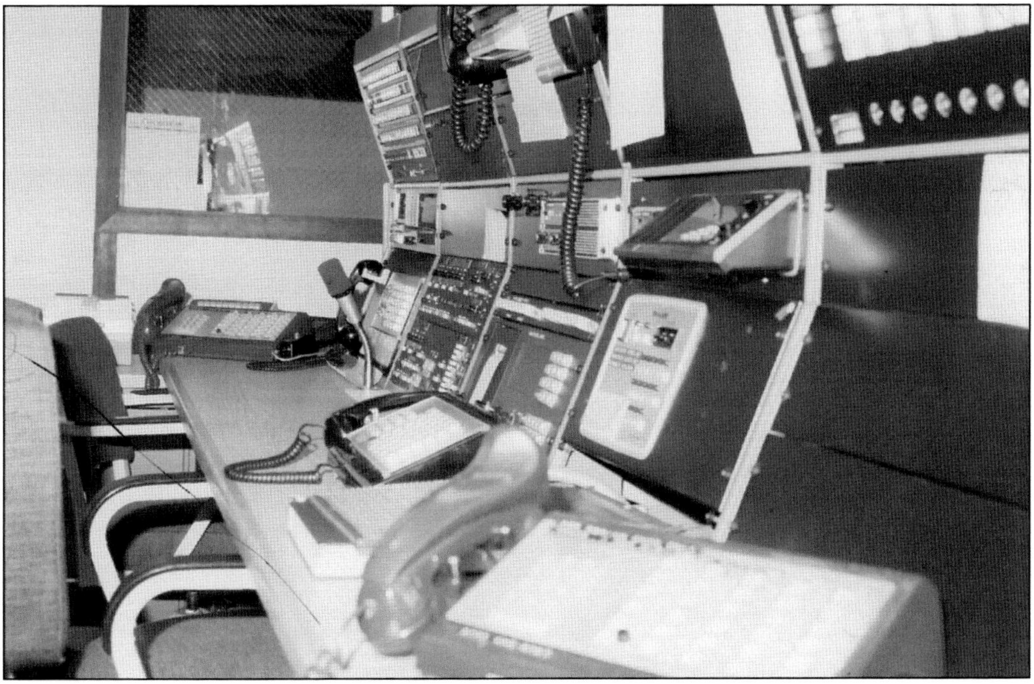

The Groton Emergency Communications Center—pictured here in 1981—serves 43,600 residents across 36 square miles. Beside the fire departments and ambulance services, it grew to include dispatch for the Lawrence + Memorial Hospital paramedics and serves as a control point for ambulance and hospital communications. (Joe Baril.)

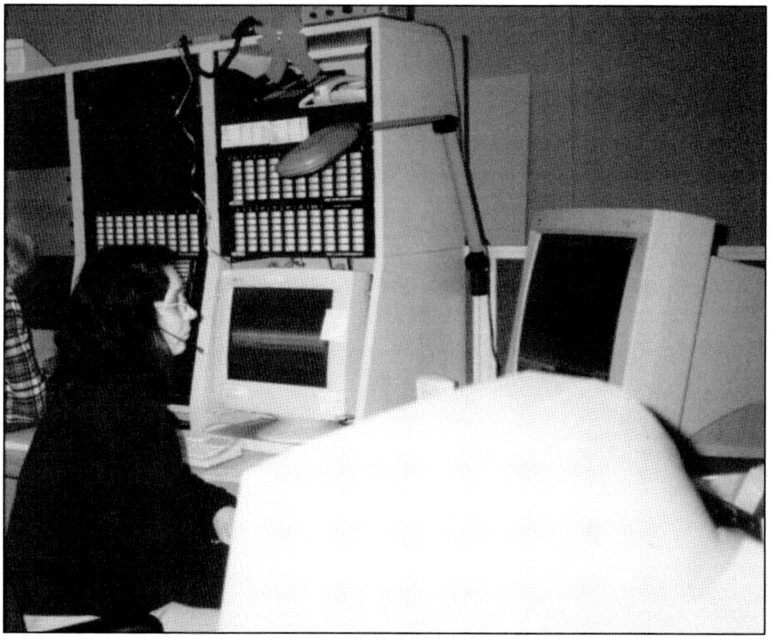

This photograph shows dispatcher Cindy Grant at work at a dispatch station at the Groton Emergency Communications Center. The center, which is located in the Town of Groton Police headquarters building, was established in 1981. (Dinah Girardi.)

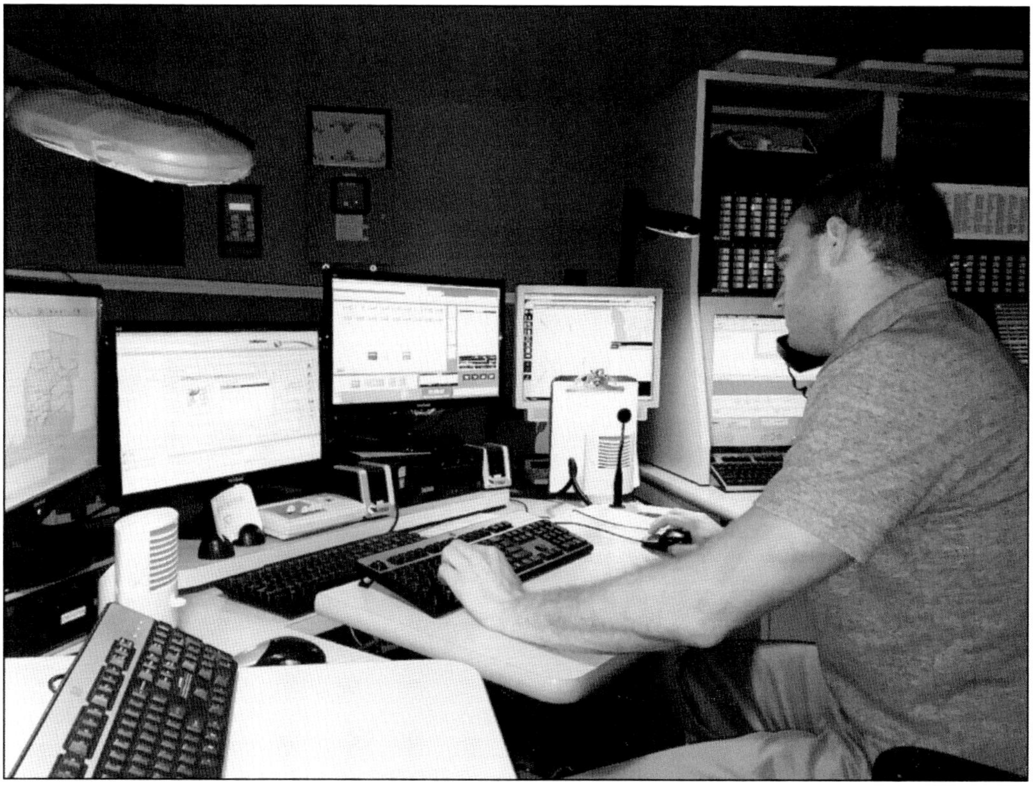

Through the years, Groton Emergency Communications Center has grown and has upgraded their equipment; computers are now the central part of the operation. With this new equipment, the dispatchers provide a vital service as the first link in the chain of emergency services. (Groton Emergency Communications Center.)

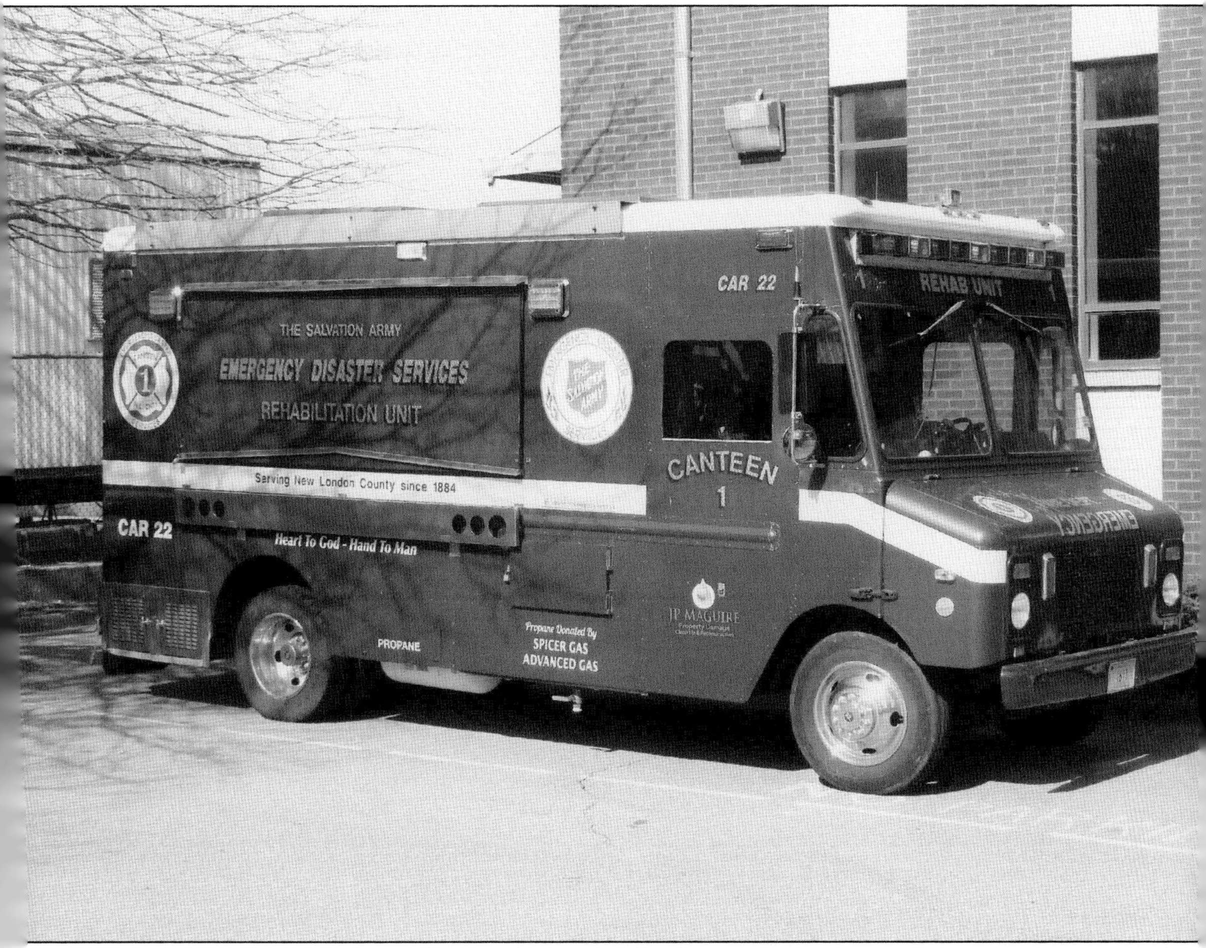

We would like to extend our appreciation to the Salvation Army's Emergency Disaster Services Rehabilitation Unit (otherwise known as the Canteen). This unit provides a much-needed service to New London County and has always supported the fire and police departments, particularly when they are operating in extreme weather conditions. The Canteen provides hot or cold drinks and snacks that are appreciated when emergency services personnel have been subjected to hot or cold weather for an extended period of time. As a way of thanking the Salvation Army for providing this service, the authors are donating the royalties from this book to the Salvation Army to support the Canteen Unit. (William Tischer.)